THE OPIOID CRISIS WAKE-UP CALL

HEALTH CARE IS STEALING THE AMERICAN DREAM. HERE'S HOW WE TAKE IT BACK.

Dave Chase

THE OPIOID CRISIS WAKE-UP CALL-HEALTH CARE IS STEALING THE AMERICAN DREAM. HERE'S HOW WE TAKE IT BACK.
www.healthrosetta.org

This book's content significantly overlaps, updates, and expands on content first published in the author's last book, The CEO's Guide to Restoring the American Dream. This book's purpose is to connect the concepts introduced in that book to the human and societal damage caused by the Opioid Crisis, as well as make the content relevant to a wider audience.

ISBN:
978-0-9992343-3-4 (Softcover)
978-0-9992343-4-1 (Hardcover)
978-0-9992343-5-8 (E-Book)

Printed primarily in the United States of America

Publisher's Cataloging-in-Publication Data
    The Opioid Crisis Wake-Up Call
    Health Care is Stealing the American Dream. Here's How We Take it Back.

    Dave Chase
        1. Health insurance—United States—Costs.
        2. Business & Economics—Insurance—Health.
        3. Employee—Medical Care—United States—Cost Control.
        4. Employer Health Care Benefits.
        5. Business & Economics—Management.

Dedicated to my family - Coleen, Abby & Cam - who have supported my never-ending passion for reforming health care, and especially to my parents - Barbara & Vern - inspiring role models who have won the Citizens of the Year award in two different towns. Thank you for being exceptional examples of how to positively impact every community you touch.

TABLE OF CONTENTS

PREFACE

By the time I was 35, I had lost ten close friends who were my age or younger. It's a gut punch to be reminded how short our time here is, but one loss hit me harder than any other: a friend died of cancer, and the system failed her in every way. She was a talented tech executive and worked her way to the top levels of Silicon Valley. She should have had access to great health care, but got a harmful treatment plan which led her to be financially, physically, and emotionally ruined leaving her 10-year-old daughter behind. It was devastating to witness.

Her death struck me particularly deeply because I realized I was part of the system. I was raised to know that if you see a wrong and don't do anything about it, you are complicit. I had started my career consulting with faith-based and children's hospitals as a revenue cycle consultant—a fancy term for generating as big a bill as possible, getting it out as fast as possible, and getting it paid as quickly as possible. At one time, this was simply to ensure that a hospital didn't forget to bill for something, but it became the root of a scheme that is arbitrary, abusive, and has absolutely devastated the working and middle class in America. Like my friend before her death, hundreds of thousands of victims of our corrupt health care system file for bankruptcy every year—even though 70% of them have insurance. I saw the fear in my friend's eyes thinking about her daughter's future, knowing that even after working hard and being extremely successful, she wasn't going to be able to leave her with much, if anything.

Not long before my friend's passing, I had been leading the most successful technology platform in health care. I was excited about how patients and doctors could finally realize value from easy-to-use software after decades of mainframe computers. But despite breakthrough technologies that could improve patient outcomes, that's not what hospitals wanted to buy. All they wanted were systems tuned to game every reimbursement opportunity the industry had to offer. Despite being at the top of my game in health care, I couldn't be party to that and vowed I wasn't going to work on technology that I knew was going to do more harm than good. I was frustrated that I didn't have the solution, so I left health care for over a decade.

Around the time I was returning to health care, a high school kid asked me to buy a candy bar for her school fundraiser. Great, I said, were they raising money for a band trip? No. It turned out they were raising money for science lab supplies. What?! Taxes paid for that stuff when I was a kid.

Turns out this often isn't the case anymore, primarily because of health care. Bill Gates devoted an entire TED talk to how health care has been devastating education: larger class sizes, laid off teachers, fewer music and arts classes, and increased college tuition for state universities and community colleges. He also outlined how devastated education budgets would impact the future by preventing bold experiments and limiting opportunities for excellence. When Gates gave his talk, California alone owed more than $60 billion in health benefits costs that it couldn't pay. I started my K-12 education in California at a time when the state was generally considered to have the best education system in the country; today it has the lowest high school graduation rates in the entire country--and the highest student to teacher ratio.[1]

The scale of the medical and financial devastation that health care has wrought on America is something most people can't imagine. The opioid crisis, the largest U.S. public health crisis in 100 years, is entirely a self-inflicted wound, driven almost entirely by a dysfunctional health care system. More than two decades of wage stagnation and decline are overwhelmingly driven by health care's hyperinflation. Today, 60 percent of the workforce makes $20/hour or less, while health insurance premiums for a family of four are over $20,000 per year. With over half of the workforce having a deductible greater than $1,000, most Americans are a bad stubbed toe away from financial ruin. And these are the people who have insurance!

Despite this gloom, I've found real hope in the solutions I've discovered. Every structural solution to prevent what happened to my friend and countless others has already been invented and proven, and is working someplace in this country. A small hotel company has the best benefits package of any employer I've ever seen—and they spend 55 percent less than employers of similar size. In addition to providing quality, affordable health care to employees and their families, they've invested a small fraction of what they saved into the local community and school system, which are seeing stunning results: crime has gone down by 67 percent and high school graduation rates have doubled to essentially 100 percent. It sounds unbelievable, but it's true, and it's happening in Orlando right now.

The most amazing discovery I've made in studying successful innovations is that the best way to slash costs is to *improve* health benefits and outcomes. How could I *not* share this great news?

The excitement from health care professionals, elected officials, employers, and other civic-minded Americans is contagious. If you've picked up this book, you are part of the solution. No matter who or where you are, you can join this effort to catalyze change and restore both hope and health to the community where you live and work.

There's no time to lose. As bad as the opioid crisis is, in its shadow are lurking other potential crises that could grow as big. While in Boston recently, not far from "Methadone Mile," I saw two things that we now know are profoundly connected— gleaming billion-dollar medical towers and students "on strike" because of school underfunding. The antidotes to both of these issues already exist. For example, we can go a long way to stopping the opioid crisis in its tracks while fixing education under-funding and preventing other potential crises through access to great value-based primary care, a critical foundation for a fair, rational, affordable, and effective health care system.

There are many things you can do to foster such a system. For example, work to ensure that your company, union, or community has access to great primary care. Implement the 12 antidotes to the opioid crisis in this book. Join the Health Rosetta community to share your successes and learn from those of others. If you are a city leader who makes health care-related decisions, lead by example with city employees and use your bully pulpit to reinvent health care in your community. If you are a union leader, follow the example of dozens of school districts around the Pittsburgh area, where labor and management leaders put aside old differences to work together for benefits that boost the health—and bottom line—of all parties.

Write down every organization you have influence over and share with them that the best way to slash health care costs is to *improve* health benefits. Share this book with them—we've made a free download available of it and my last book (*CEO's Guide to Restoring the American Dream*) at www.healthrosetta.org/friends. We care more about spreading success than losing a few book sales. Whatever your role, start with one organization and one tactic.

For too long, we've let health care crush the American Dream. We can't take another 20 years of economic depression for the working and middle class. Whether we knew it or not, we all contributed to this mess. Now, it's on us to fix it. When change happens community by community, it's impossible to stop. Yes, health care stole the American Dream. But, it's absolutely possible to take it back. Join us to make it happen in your community.

INTRODUCTION

The opioid crisis is America's largest public health crisis in 100 years, a self-inflicted wound caused by a catastrophically dysfunctional health care system featuring ill-designed health benefits and employers who are unwitting enablers. Fortunately, upstream solutions involving those same employers, along with civil leaders and organizations, have been created and proven. It's time to broaden their application and stop the crisis in its tracks—and, with it, the system that has bankrupted so many families and communities.

This book won't rehash the details of the rise of the opioid crisis. You can't beat *Dreamland* by Sam Quinones for a compelling narrative of the parallel rise in prescription opioids and street opioids such as heroin and fentanyl. Likewise, if you want a public policy paper on the opioid crisis as well as how best to address those *already* enslaved by opioid use disorders, *Confronting Our Nation's Opioid Crisis* by the Aspen Health Strategy Group[2] is outstanding. We have included in the appendix a table of the evidenced-based approaches to address those already suffering from opioid use disorders.

The objective of this book is to focus on what can be done *today* by civic leaders, whether they are mayors and other elected officials, union leaders, social service and faith-based organizations as well as civic-minded business leaders to go upstream and avoid enabling more waves of addiction. After all, the crisis can't be solved if the flow of new opioid overuse disorders isn't stopped in its tracks. As we'll discuss later, the opioid crisis is a microcosm of the even larger health care crisis providing a catalyst for communities to pull together across social and political boundaries. So, we'll pull back to look at how the opioid crisis fits into the broad-based negative impact that the status quo health care system has wrought on the American Dream.

The U.S. working and middle classes have gone backwards financially in the last 20 years and the culprit is our health care system. This was the conclusion of a groundbreaking 2013 RAND study, which found that:[3]

- Health care expenditures, including insurance premiums, out-of-pocket expenditures, and taxes devoted to health care, nearly doubled between 1999 and 2009.
- This increase substantially eroded what an average family must spend on everything else, leaving them with only $95 more per month than in 2007.
- Had health care costs paralleled the Consumer Price Index, rather than outpacing it, an average American family would have had an additional $450 per month—more than $5,000 per year—to spend on other priorities.

If the situation is dire, it is anything but hopeless. I've seen all kinds of communities, organizations, and companies—large and small, public and private, rural and urban—turn things around by rejecting the status quo and improving health benefits, which turns out to be the best way to cut costs and cut opioid abuse down to size. You can do the same. This book will show you how and get you started down the path.

The first step is the most important and the hardest: to accept that you can contribute to transforming health in your community. Whether you are an organization leader, a civic leader, a member of your child's PTA, part of a faith-based or social service organization, or an employer, making this shift in mindset will benefit you, your community, organizations you are part of, and, by extension, your country. Here are three good reasons to make the shift and follow through:

1. **Help save our country and communities** – As we'll discuss in more detail, the opioid crisis and waste in health care's status quo are running our country off a cliff. It's a major contributor to personal bankruptcies, broken public budgets, wage stagnation, and much more. If we don't make the shift, health care could consume essentially all household income in less than 20 years.
2. **Reinvest resources previously squandered in health care on true well-being** – Our kids' future, our incomes, and community resilience have been stolen by an under-performing health care system. Communities such as Pittsburgh have shown how not squandering money on ineffective and even harmful health care can mean smaller class sizes, more librarians, and better pay and benefits for teachers. Private employers reinvesting a portion of what they save have seen dramatic decreases in crime and spikes in high school graduation rates.
3. **Foster economic development by making health care local again** – Economic Development 3.0 brings the "shop local" concept back to health care. This is key, because roughly half of health care spending currently leaves the local economy, even though there are few things more local than going to your doctor. Given that health care is roughly one-fifth of the economy, keeping that spent close to home can be a tremendous economic boost for communities.

Just in case you're still not persuaded, let's go negative for a second. Given that millennials will see half to two-thirds of their lifetime earnings going to health care if we don't change the status quo trajectory, civil unrest could become a distinct possibility.

The good news is that making the shift in your mind and acting on it delivers 100 percent of the time. There are many examples to show the way. Let's get started.

A NOTE ON READING THIS BOOK

The first two sections of this book, *The Current Situation* and *How and Why Wages Have Been Flat for Over 20 Years,* explore in detail the case presented in this introduction, helping you understand specifically what has gone wrong with health care and what the consequences for our employees, organizations, communities, and country.

The last two sections, *Doing It Right* and *The Future: Health Rosetta Guides Us to the Health 3.0 Vision,* will take you step by step through key solutions you can start implementing immediately. We draw on individual successes at specific organizations as well as big picture systemic change. Case studies are scattered throughout.

Since virtually every city in America is struggling with the economic consequences of the out-of-control health care system and the human toll of the opioid crisis, I'd draw your attention to three chapters designed to help civic leaders turn the situation around: Chapter 18: Economic Development 3.0 – Communities Take Center Stage, Chapter 19: Mayors Must Lead Cities out of the Opioid Crisis, and Chapter 19: Making Sure Opioid Mitigation Plans Mitigate the Right Things. The last of these chapters recognizes that hundreds of cities, counties, and states have filed suits to recover the externalized costs of the opioid crisis. We curated insights from many of the nation's experts on the underlying drivers of the crisis to come up with the key pillars of an effective settlement that recognizes that opioid abuse is emblematic of a much larger problem. Feel free to jump around. Each chapter generally stands on its own.

For readers of my previous book, the *CEO's Guide To Restoring The American Dream*, this book serves as the follow-on edition. The framing is around the opioid crisis being emblematic of the larger health care dysfunction. This edition is also designed to a reach a broader audience to include civic leaders ranging from mayors to union leaders to faith and social service leaders to police and fire chiefs. I have also added key take-aways for each chapter and there's references to more case studies of various organizations having success transforming health in our communities. To expedite your reading, the following chapters are new:

- Preface - Why I wrote the book and why there's an urgent imperative to tackle the crisis
- Introduction - Context for how the opioid crisis is a microcosm of the larger health care dysfunction
- Chapter 1: The Opioid Crisis Isn't an Anomaly
- Chapter 16: The Future of Health Will Be Local, Open, and Independent
- Chapter 17: Health 3.0 Vision and Implications For Providers & Government
- Chapter 18: Economic Development 3.0: Communities Take Center Stage

To learn more, read on or visit healthrosetta.org
What is the Health Rosetta? The blueprint for evidence-based health purchasing. It's a practical approach built on what successful purchasers do.

For ongoing insight, best practices, and updates, join the Health Rosetta newsletter at healthrosetta.org/employers. Throughout the book, I have a variety of email addresses to send to related to particular chapters. However, if you have success stories of how communities are being rebuilt, have general ideas or feedback, email me at dave.chase@ healthrosetta.org.

A Word about Words

Health care always seems to use ten different words for essentially the same thing, each with some supposed slight variation in meaning that isn't even consistently used by those of us in the industry. I have also included terms that may be unfamiliar to those outside the health benefits profession. To minimize confusion, I have tried to use consistent terminology, as follows.

- **Benefits broker, consultant, and advisor.** These three terms are often used interchangeably in the real world to refer to people who arrange, negotiate, and/or purchase a health plan on behalf of a third party. I use *broker* to signify a person who operates under the status quo, taking a highly conflicted approach to purchasing health benefits. I use *advisor* or *consultant* to signify someone operating under the modern, high-value, transparent approach.
- **ERISA.** The Employee Retirement Income Security Act of 1974 is a federal law that sets minimum standards for most voluntarily established pension and health plans in private industry to provide protection for individuals in these plans.
- **Health plan.** This refers to a specific health benefits plan, whether fully insured or self-insured.
- **Insurance company or carrier.** These refer to the organizations that provide insurance and/or self-insured plan administration services
- **PBM.** Pharmacy Benefit Manager is a Third-Party Administrator (TPA) of prescription drug programs for commercial health plans, self-insured employer plans, Medicare Part D plans, the Federal Employees Health Benefits Program, and state government employee plans.
- **People.** I use a couple of different terms depending on context. *Individual* is the default. *Patient* is for people

receiving care. *Member* or *employee* refer to individuals from a health plan or employer's perspective.

- **Plan administrator.** This is the organization that performs the noninsurance pieces of a health plan, like claims adjudication. It includes Administrative Services Organizations (ASO) tied to insurance companies and independent Third-Party Administrators (TPA).
- **Provider organization and clinician.** These terms cover the people and entities that provide health care services. This includes physicians, nurses, hospitals, health systems, and other providers of health care services.
- **Quadruple Aim.** Refers to the simultaneous pursuit of improving the care team experience (both professional and non-professional members of the care team), patient experience of care, improving the health of populations, and reducing the per capita cost of health care.
- **Self-insured or self-funded.** These are organizations that may use an insurance company provider network, however they pay the claims and take on the financial risk. Typically, organizations over 100 employees are self-insured, however they have stop-loss policies.
- **Stop-Loss Insurance.** All but the largest employers have stop loss policies that cover unpredictable claims such as cancer, organ transplants and other outlier claims.
- **TPA- Third-Party Administrators.** Self-insured organizations normally use an independent third party to administer health claims. A variant of this are Administrative Services Only (ASO) organizations that are owned by insurance carriers with the resulting pros and cons laid out Part III.
- **Workplace wellness program.** The term *wellness* has been co-opted by a large industry of vendors that largely sells products with no or negative ROI. I use this more specific term to refer to these programs.

Part I

The Current Situation

*M*ost explanations of the opioid crisis are greatly oversimplified, leading to "solutions" that are ineffective at best and inflict immense damage on the American people and the American economy at worst. This is because, tragically, the opioid crisis isn't an anomaly. Rather, it's the logical byproduct of a catastrophically dysfunctional health care system.

While it's hardly breaking news that there are problems in health care, the extent of the collateral damage—of which opioid abuse is just one example—is less well known. This section of the book goes beyond the visible parts of our present system to explore the underlying dynamics and perverse incentives behind many of the problems.

The good news is that, despite what you've heard, we already have fixes for most of the root causes of health care's dysfunction, fixes that can prevent disasters such as the opioid abuse epidemic from arising in the first place, or at least greatly reduce their damage. We simply have to get the word out. Millennials will make this happen. They are now the largest generation in history and the largest chunk of the workforce. They're changing our world in ways that hold great promise for health care.

CHAPTER 1

THE OPIOID CRISIS ISN'T AN ANOMALY

"No one is immune to addiction; it afflicts people of all ages, races, classes, and professions." – Patrick J. Kennedy

For 37 years, Tom L. Shupe, a senior manager at an Oklahoma manufacturer, has been on the frontlines of the challenges facing U.S. manufacturing. He's full of insights, but the most surprising one is that he blames substance abuse—specifically opioids—for most of these challenges. "It's all addiction issues," says Shupe. He calls the opioid crisis, which is really an epidemic of addiction, "probably the biggest threat in manufacturing, period."[7]

Here's something even more shocking: Employers are unwitting accomplices, enablers, as well as victims of the largest public health crisis since the 1918 flu epidemic. Overwhelmingly, those suffering from opioid use disorders are working age or their dependents. Through our health benefits, we have funded a self-inflicted wound that is emblematic of the even broader dysfunction pervasive in our health care system.

Let's look at just one example. A major challenge of physically demanding, hourly jobs is that if you don't work, you don't get paid. Sixty percent of the workforce makes $20 per hour or less[8]– many of them paid hourly. When an injury occurs, the worker must choose between not working (and not getting paid), or continuing to work despite the pain. Opioids start as a short-term fix, enabling the worker to stay on the job, but they also slow—and can even prevent—healing. If the worker has the predisposition to addiction, a vicious escalating cycle takes off. Jordan Barbour, director of clinical operations, psychiatry, and addiction medicine at Geisinger Health, described the common progression from addiction to work issues to job loss to street drugs, incarceration, and Hepatitis C, all costing their family and community dearly.

Beyond the obvious human toll, there is a financial imperative to solve this crisis. Supporting early identification of addiction, along with access to effective treatment and relapse prevention, doesn't just help the sick and suffering. It makes great *economic* sense.

Make no mistake: The opioid crisis is a complicated issue over 30 years in the making. But companies have played a major role in creating and sustaining the crisis. And a vanguard of employers are realizing that they have a major role to play in solving it, and that the solutions fall well beyond what the government alone can do. In this, the epidemic is a microcosm and mirror of our failing health care system as a whole; ending it will move us meaningfully down the path toward solving the larger crisis.

There is a growing trend that equates people suffering from chronic pain with people suffering from opioid addiction. In fact, there is an array of rare diseases, such as Ehlers–Danlos syndrome, where well-managed opioid regimens can be the appropriate course of treatment. We must be careful that the zeal to address the opioid abuse doesn't inflict unnecessary suffering on those with chronic pain. This is where having adequate time to treat patients as individuals is imperative; other countries manage to work with these long-term patients without triggering an opioid crisis.

Primary Drivers

There are 12 primary drivers of the opioid crisis, all of which must be addressed by the country and, specifically, by employers.

1. *Undertreated pain leading to a 5th vital sign and increased prescribing*

This concept was initially promoted by the American Pain Society to elevate awareness of pain treatment among health care professionals. The Veteran's Health Administration made pain a 5th vital sign in 1998, followed by their creation of the "Pain as the 5th Vital Sign Toolkit" in 2000. This made pain equal to things like blood pressure—a number to be managed with medications or lifestyle changes. In 2001, the Joint Commission established standards for pain assessment and treatment in response to the national outcry about widespread undertreatment, putting severe pressure on doctors and nurses to prescribe opioids.

2. *Pharmaceutical industry sales and marketing blitz*

Pharmaceutical companies capitalized on the other drivers listed here. Through major marketing campaigns,[4] they got physicians to prescribe opioid products such as OxyContin and Vicodin and in high quantities—even though the evidence[5] of their efficacy treating chronic pain is very weak[6] , and the evidence that they cause harm in the long term is very strong[7] . Perhaps no organizations had more ability to flag the growing crisis than pharmacy benefits managers and distributors, as they had the complete view of dramatic increases in opioid volume; instead, they let the crisis explode in severity.

In contrast to other countries, U.S. physicians stopped prescribing slow and low, one byproduct of which is huge amounts of opioids readily available in medicine cabinets for people suffering any level of pain—and for teenagers to abuse. Direct-to-consumer advertising also significantly increased patient requests for opioid prescriptions.[8]

3. Opioids used for non-cancer chronic pain (e.g., back pain)

Eighty percent of people will have lower back pain in their life-time, making it one of the most common reasons for missing work[9]. Stress or inappropriate posture, a sedentary lifestyle, and poor workplace ergonomics can all lead to back, neck, and other kinds of musculoskeletal (MSK) pain. The American Academy of Neurology (AAN) told its members that the risks of opioids in the treatment of noncancer chronic pain patients far outweighed the benefits, yet the practice is widespread. The AAN observed that if physicians stopped using the drugs to treat conditions such as fibromyalgia, back pain, and headache, long-term exposure to opioids could decline by as much as 50 percent.

4. Economic distress

Drug, alcohol, and suicide mortality rates are higher in counties with more economic distress and a larger working class. Many counties with high mortality rates have also seen significant manufacturing employment losses over the past several decades[10]. For every one percent rise in unemployment, there's a four percent rise in addiction and a seven percent increase in emergency department visits.[11] Remember, health care costs can consume as much as 50 percent of the total compensation package for people making less than $15 per hour[12], suppressing wages and holding back job growth.

5. Declining reimbursement that increases physician prescribing of opioids

Reimbursement for physicians in private practice continues to decline, despite an escalation of both operating costs and adminis-trative burden. As patient volume increases to make up for lower payment, the average amount of time a provider can spend with the patient decreases, boosting the probability of the provider writing a prescription[13]. The pressures to increase volume make it incredibly challenging for most providers, who typically are not well versed in addiction medicine, to identify and effectively manage patients with chronic pain and potentially undiagnosed substance abuse.

6. Insurers' refusal to cover validated treatments

Insurance companies' refusal to cover scientifically validated approaches for pain management such as physical therapy (PT), cognitive behavior therapy, psychological support, or interventional pain procedures also contributed to this crisis. Mental health parity legislation forced insurers' hands when it took effect in 2010, but PT and workplace redesign continue to be marginalized despite their proven effects. Even when a physician appeals to an insurance company to approve treatments that may help the patient, several months or even years can go by, especially in worker's compensation cases[14]. By then, the patient may be on escalating doses of opioids just to function as a result of increased tolerance. This results in more anxiety and depression, and can often lead to financial devastation from loss of employment.

7. Health-related state/local budget challenges that weaken community resilience

Governments can only raise taxes so much. We've seen how out-of-control health care costs have eaten away at the very items that make a community more resistant to public health challenges; every budget item that has been cut could help stem the opioid crisis. One example is mental health funding, a particularly powerful antidote to the opioid crisis. At the local level, funding shortfalls are exacerbated as tax-exempt health systems are often among the largest property owners, yet pay no taxes. And still America's perverse health care incentives reinforce the misconception that building hospitals is a long-term economic driver.

8. Mental disorders treated with opioids

According to a recent study, more than half of all opioid prescriptions in the United States annually go to adults with a mental illness, who represent just 16 percent of the U.S. population[15].

It's important to note that depression and anxiety worsen pain and vice versa. Healthy and effective stress and life-coping skills, available through a value-based primary care model, can decrease the impact of this pain.

9. Patient satisfaction scores' influence on hospital income

Results from HCAHPS and Press Ganey patient satisfaction surveys, which directly impact hospital income, further amped up the pressure. Administrators harangued nurses and doctors to make patients happy by giving them opioids. Data from approximately 52,000 adults was assessed from 2000 to 2007 via the Medical Expenditure Panel Survey; a 26 percent increase in mortality rates was observed among those who were most satisfied[16]. CMS announced it will remove pain management from its determination of hospital payments beginning in 2018, but that doesn't undo the damage that has been done.

10. Patients looking for a quick fix

An unfortunate part of American culture is seeking quick fixes. Patients want a pill for instant pain relief and advertising has conditioned them to expect one. This tendency is exacerbated by doctors looking for a quick fix during their short appointments with patients. The reality is that most patients hear more from pharmaceutical companies (16-18 hours of pharma ads per year[17]) than from their doctor (typically under 2 hours per year).

With this "instant-fix" conditioning from players across the health care system, many patients aren't willing to invest time in cognitive behavioral therapy, mindful meditation, or a regular program of PT/exercise. At the same time, we've forgotten that some pain is a good indicator of a problem to solve and shouldn't be instantly numbed.

11. Lack of access to specialists

In many rural areas, availability of PT and mental health treatment can be limited and pain specialists trained in non-opioid pain management are shockingly rare. Consequently, the only tool in the toolbox has been more pills.

12. *Criminal abuse of the system*

In many places, doctors lacking ethics were easier to find than proper pain treatment. Initially, "pill mills" disguised as "pain clinics" gave legitimate pain doctors a bad name. Pharmacy benefits managers and pharmacies were more than willing to go along with the game, making billions in the process. The public and private sector purchasers dropped the ball on this by not having opiate prescribing databases in place to catch the bad actors. As prescription opioid availability tightened up, cheap black tar heroin filled the need for individuals suffering from addiction; people addicted to opioid medications are 40 times more likely to get addicted to heroin.[18]

Let's clear up one misunderstanding: The vast majority of doctors, even those who are salaried employees, have no financial incentive to get their patients hooked. They simply want their patients to get better and the wait time to be seen by a pain specialist can be weeks long. A chronic pain patient who no longer needs pills or experiences pain is the best marketing a doctor could ask for. Most doctors were trying to do the right thing based on what they knew about opioids at the time and what insurers would cover.

A Weight Around Employers' Necks

Before delving into the antidotes, let's take a quick look at the damage opioids are wreaking on the American economy in general and employers in particular.

Here's a good starting point: Opioid overdoses—often in conjunction with other central nervous system depressant drugs like benzodiazepines or alcohol—are now the leading cause of death for working people under 50 years old, surpassing deaths from guns and car crashes.[19]

LinkedIn's Work in Progress podcast looked at the negative impact of the opioid crisis on employers[20]. There were a couple big takeaways:

- At a Congressional hearing focused on opioids and their economic consequences, Ohio attorney general Mike DeWine estimated that 40 percent of job applicants in the state either failed or refused a drug test[21]. The result: In certain places, solid middle-class jobs can't be filled. In Congressional testimony earlier in July 2017, Federal Reserve chair Janet Yellen connected opioid use to a decline in the labor participation rate.
- The issue is amplifying labor shortages in industries like trucking, which has had difficulty for the last six years finding qualified workers. It's also pushing employers to broaden their job searches, recruiting people from greater distances. The issue is not just workplace safety and productivity, but whether workplaces need humans at all. Some manufacturers claim opioids are forcing them to automate faster.

Some may find drug testing intrusive, but many jobs—whether in manufacturing or other sectors such as transportation—pose potentially huge consequences from accidents. You may not recall that opioids were to blame for the Staten Island Ferry disaster that killed 11 and injured scores[22] . A very big problem for employers is "presenteeism," where an employee performs sub-optimally, often as a result of impairing pain or medications, especially opioids. Unlike cocaine or heroin, where a confirmatory drug screen results in termination, a "legitimate" prescription for oxycodone and Xanax is a much murkier problem.

The *New York Times* reported that workers who received high doses of opioid painkillers to treat injuries like back strain stayed off the job three times longer than those with similar injuries who took lower doses.[23] When disability and medical care payments are combined, the cost of a workplace injury is nine times higher when a strong narcotic like OxyContin is used. The sum of an employee's medical expenses and lost wage payments is about $13,000, but when he or she is prescribed a short-acting painkiller like Percocet, that figure triples to $39,000—and triples again to $117,000 when a stronger, longer-acting opioid like OxyContin is prescribed.

Insurers' policies of covering painkillers but not evidence-based PT approaches may "have created a monster," said Dr. Bernyce M. Peplowski, the medical director of the State Compensation Insurance Fund of California.

It's Not Just Opioids

Cathryn Jakobson Ramin devoted an entire book (*Crooked: Outwitting the Back Pain Industry and Getting on the Road to Recovery*) to how little evidence informs our back pain industry. And opioids aren't the only class of medication that is being inappropriately prescribed. Benzodiazepines, or benzos, comprise a class of depressants that most people know by the brand names Ativan, Klonopin, Valium, and Xanax. These medications are typically used to treat anxiety, insomnia, and seizures. And they're being prescribed at alarmingly high rates.

Prescriptions for benzodiazepines more than tripled, and fatal overdoses more than quadrupled between 1996 and 2013[24]. In fact, benzos have been so grossly overused that they are among not only the top-prescribed psychiatric medications[25] but also the most prescribed medications of any type in the United States.

Like other interventions such as non-evidence-based opioid prescriptions and spinal procedures, benefits of benzos have been oversold. For decades, they've been prescribed for anxiety and sleep, but the evidence indicates that they don't work very well, and they are not intended for long-term use.[26]

The Path Forward

While we must be smarter about treating those already afflicted with opioid addictions, we must also turn off the spigot to clean up the mess. The silver lining of the opioid crisis is that it shines a light on just how abysmally our health care system has been performing. True health starts at home and in our communities, not in hospitals or in pills.

At the end of Sam Quinones's gripping book on the opioid crisis, *Dreamland,* he argues that the sustainable fix is "a community that addresses social determinants of health like safe neighborhoods, quality jobs, and a health care system that can treat those afflicted with opioid use disorders while preventing others from being drawn into the hell of addiction." Employers using the opioid crisis as a catalyst to change their approach to health care can do a great service by revitalizing the broader community. By extension, a growing employer has a better pool of prospective employees to draw on.

Put simply, employers who adopt Health Rosetta-type benefits programs are far more likely to have much lower rates of employees and dependents suffering from opiate use disorders. Given that the opioid crisis isn't an outlier situation but a microcosm of a larger dysfunction, it's clear how solving one of the largest public health crises in American history can serve as a catalyst for dramatically improving our entire health care system. Let's revisit our 12 drivers with this in mind, drawing on examples provided elsewhere in the book. (More details are provided on the Health Rosetta website.) See the listed chapters for explanations of unfamiliar terms and concepts.

Note that the antidotes listed below are focused on upstream prevention. For those already suffering from opioid use disorders, it's critical that health plans cover the best evidence-based treatments (see Appendix A for a list of evidence-based approaches). Today, that means medication-assisted therapy, although the field of study is evolving, so it's critical plans reflect the latest developments.

Opioid crisis driver	Proven employer antidotes
Undertreated pain leading to a 5th vital sign	Value-based primary care is critical to physicians understanding the issues behind a patient's pain: With MSK-related costs accounting for 20 percent of health care spending, wise employers integrate PT specialists into primary care and workplace design and seek out organizations that use PT upfront in triage. (*Case Study: City of Milwaukee*)
	Appropriate use of drug testing and regular checks of state prescription drug monitoring reports can help identify a substance use disorder and start the process to wellness earlier.
	(*Chapter 21 – Value-Based Primary Care; Case Study: Rosen Hotel & Resorts*)
Big pharma's sales and marketing blitz	Let's face it, sales and marketing works. Value-based primary care organizations ensure clinicians receive education on—and have in place—viable, quantifiable treatment options that maximize value and come from unbiased sources—and have time to explain to patients how non-opioid treatment options are more effective.
	(*Chapter 13 – The 7 Habits of Highly Effective Benefits Professionals; Chapter 15 – Independent Claims Administrators Vs. Insurance Company Claims Administrators – The Trade-Offs; Case Study: Langdale Industries*)
Opioids used for non-cancer chronic pain (e.g., back pain)	Progressive benefits programs weave non-opioid options into both clinic and non-clinic settings. One example is PT for back pain. Another is Rosen Hotel's incorporating movement training and ergonomic adjustments into the workplace.
	A well-informed health plan document should include policies spelling out certain steps to be taken before and after administration of opioids, placing a time limit on how long an employee can be authorized to take the medication.
	(*Chapter 7 – 7 Tricks Used to Redistribute Money From Your Organization to the Health Care Industry; Chapter 11 – You Run a Health Care Business Whether You Like it or Not; Chapter 12 – How to Pick a Benefits Consultant, Chapter 14 – Centers of Excellence Offer a Golden Opportunity; Case Study: Rosen Hotel & Resorts*)

Economic distress	The case study about Tulsa-based Enovation Controls shows how a manufacturer with a blue-collar workforce designed benefits that make smart decisions free (e.g., eliminating copays and deductibles when using high-value surgical hospitals) and bad decisions expensive (e.g., going to low-quality providers who have higher complication rates, poor outcomes, and overtreatment).
	With poor plan design, more than half the workforce is one minor medical issue away from financial ruin. Wise plan design eliminates cost-sharing for smart health care decisions. Increasingly, employers such as the city of Kirkland and Palmer Johnson Power Systems put more money in employees' pockets by educating and engaging them in wise health care decisions.
	(Case Study: Enovation Controls)
Declining reimbursement that increases physician prescribing of opioids	In a value-based primary care model, patients have the proper amount of time with their doctor. An increase in patient interaction time shuts down some of the on-ramp to opioids, whether it's inappropriate opioid prescribing or unnecessary and excessive surgeries that are typically followed by opioid prescriptions.
	(Chapter 15 – Independent Claims Administrators Vs. Insurance Company Claims Administrators – The Trade-Offs)
Insurers' refusal to cover validated treatments	Health Rosetta-type plans outlined in Part IV pay for evidence-based services, e.g., cognitive behavioral therapy, PT, behavioral health services delivered via telehealth, value-based primary care, etc.
	(Chapter 3 – America Has Gone to War For Far Less; Chapter 7 – 7 Tricks Used to Redistribute Money From Your Organization to the Health Care Industry; Chapter 14 – Centers of Excellence Offer a Golden Opportunity; Chapter 15 – Independent Claims Administrators Vs. Insurance Company Claims Administrators – The Trade-Offs)

Health-related state/local budget challenges that weaken community resilience	Examples abound in our case studies. On the East coast, the Pittsburgh schools' case study shows how avoiding squandering dollars by steering school district employees and dependents away from low-value (if high reputation) medical centers can translate into better teacher pay and smaller class sizes. The city of Milwaukee has avoided many budget struggles afflicting other large Midwestern cities by controlling health care costs. On the West coast, the city of Kirkland (WA) has also found that the best way to slash health care costs is to *improve* benefits.[27] While many communities are pulling back on investments that drive health outcomes (e.g., walkability, safety, parks, clean air/water), Kirkland is able to maintain or increase these investments in community well-being. *(Case Studies: Pittsburgh Schools, City of Milwaukee)*
Mental disorders treated with opioids	Evidence-based benefits plans ensure behavioral health is woven into primary care and isn't an afterthought. A critical success factor is removing access barriers to mental health professionals. Where there is sufficient employee concentration, behavioral health services should exist inside clinics. In other settings, it's more practical to have the mental health specialist connected remotely, an approach that also overcomes the disparity in different locations' access to mental health professionals. *(Chapter 21-Value-Based Primary Care)* Behavioral health issues are particularly short-changed in the rushed, "drive-by" appointments that are all too common in volume-driven primary care. Since mental health issues underlie so many exacerbations of chronic diseases, it is part of the "magic" of a primary care setting that there is time to pick up on issues that may keep someone from complying with a care plan. *(Chapter 15– Independent Claims Administrators Vs. Insurance Company Claims Administrators – The Trade-Offs)*

Patient satisfaction scores' influence on hospital income	Evidence is mixed on whether patient satisfaction correlates with improved outcomes—or greater inpatient use, higher overall health care and prescription drug expenditures, and increased mortality[28]. Wise employers contract with health care organizations focused on other metrics—for example, the Net Promoter Score (NPS), a measure of customer likelihood to recommend a product or service and more likely aligned with holistic approaches focused on keeping people well. While NPS scoring alone won't solve the problem, it's frequently an indicator of an organization that puts the individual, rather than revenue optimization, at the center of their design. *(Chapter 3 – America Has Gone to War For Far Less; Chapter 7 – 7 Tricks Used to Redistribute Money From Your Organization to the Health Care Industry).*
Patients looking for a quick fix	Value-based primary care organizations recognize that pain rarely has quick fixes; there is usually some issue beneath the pain—stress, ergonomics, lifestyle—and doctors need sufficient time with patients to uncover it. Volume-centric, fee-for-service primary care exacerbates the pressure on doctors to deliver a quick fix. Employers such as IBM realize that investing in proper primary care that weaves in PT and mental health not only lowers costs, also contributes to a high-performance workforce.
Lack of access to specialists	As we will see, sending employees to centers of excellence and using telemedicine are two increasingly common ways savvy companies are overcoming this problem. From both a lack of specialist access and burdensome pricing perspectives, the Langdale case study shows how it can be done—and, in the case of travel, pay for itself many times over—in rural Georgia. *(Chapter 14 – Centers of Excellence Offer a Golden Opportunity; Chapter 26 – "ERISA Fiduciary Risk is the Largest Undisclosed Risk I've Seen in My Career", Case Study: Langdale Industries).*
Criminal abuse of the system	This is mostly outside the domain of employers; however, effective approaches make employees less vulnerable to pursuing illegal drugs.

Key Take-aways

- The opioid crisis has been funded and fueled by employer-paid health benefits. Once unwitting enablers of the opioid crisis, smart employers understand the crisis can't be solved without their active engagement.
- This book highlights wise employers and smart benefit strategies that have created replicable microcosms of high-performing health care systems as good as any in the world. It's in employers' enlightened self-interest to follow suit.
- A balanced approach must be employed to solve the opioid crisis. The vast majority of public policy response to the crisis has been on addressing those already addicted. This must be balanced with stopping addiction upstream before it starts. To this day, extraordinary rates of opioid prescriptions continue in the United States – rates far exceeding other countries.

CHAPTER 2

SO HOW DID WE GET HERE

"Out, out, brief candle! Life's but a walking shadow, a poor player that struts and frets his hour upon the stage and is heard no more. It is a tale told by an idiot, full of sound and fury, signifying nothing." – Macbeth

So How Did We Get Here?

Why is health care so broken? Following the money is a good place to start. Our problems started with tax policy in the 1940s. During WWII, we had wage controls, but employer-paid benefits didn't count as wages. To attract employees, employers started offering more and more health benefits without paying attention to what these benefits cost. This is our original sin. It could also be our fount of redemption.

Today, the tax break for employer-paid benefits is estimated at over $600 billion, making it the largest tax break in the tax code, the nation's second largest entitlement after Medicare,[29] and the primary wage suppression driver.

Over time, this practice sheltered us from the true cost of the care we buy, creating enormous dysfunction in what care we pay for and how we pay for it. We ended up focusing on a certain type of high-technology, acute medical care—which we financially reward far more than lower-level preventive and chronic care—without regard for the quality of the outcomes or value of the care. Because what difference does it make? Most of us get our care paid for by our employer or a government entity, who are just as ignorant about the true costs as we are. And here's the kicker: Most physicians and hospitals don't even know what it really costs to provide care because no one has held them accountable for such a long time.

This has big consequences. Our system's financial incentives aren't aligned with the outcomes we want, which most of us define as staying healthy in the first place and receiving high quality care when we need it, while still being able to afford and live a satisfying life. Instead, over decades, our health care system has made millions of small decisions to increase the quantity of procedures and pills provided, which increases revenue, resulting in hyperinflating costs and, sometimes, devastating consequences such as the opioid crisis.

It's a sad equation: Poor financial incentives + we all want care + decades of small decisions = where we are today. The Kaiser Foundation found that "since Medicare passed, per capita [health care] spending has grown more than 50-fold. This far outstrips per capita spending on all other goods and services by at least 5 times."[30] The trend is only accelerating. Figure 1 is from the *Wall Street Journal* and shows that health care takes 25 percent more of middle-income household spending than in 2007.

The Annual Benefits Kabuki Dance

Much of this dire situation is due to what benefits expert Craig Lack calls the annual kabuki dance of employers and health plans, which he described to me in a memorable conversation. Lack, CEO of the consulting firm ENERGI and co-author of *Think and Grow Rich Today*, says employers have been led to believe the best they can hope for is merely a less bad rate increase—even though there has been little to no increase in the underlying costs of medicine.

"Every year, CFOs ask their human resources (HR) team for a budget increase target. The overburdened and risk-averse nature of HR at most organizations is to preserve the status quo. The insurance companies know this and typically come in with an increase of 11-14 percent; the insurance brokers know this and "negotiate" a less bad increase, staying below the CFO's budget, and there you have it. Check the box, health care can be put to bed. See you next year. That's what passes for health care risk management at far too many organizations."

A Bigger Bite

Middle-class families' spending on health care has increased 25% since 2007. Other basic needs, such as clothing and food, have decreased.

Percent change in middle-income households' spending on basic needs (2007 to 2014)

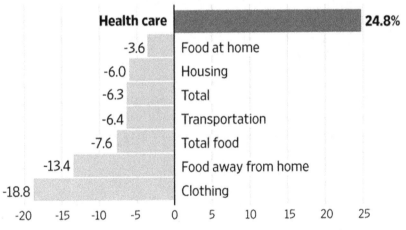

Category	Percent change
Health care	24.8%
Food at home	-3.6
Housing	-6.0
Total	-6.3
Transportation	-6.4
Total food	-7.6
Food away from home	-13.4
Clothing	-18.8

Sources: Brookings Institution analysis of Consumer Expenditure Survey, Labor Department

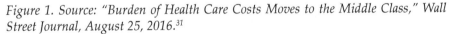

THE WALL STREET JOURNAL.

Figure 1. Source: "Burden of Health Care Costs Moves to the Middle Class," Wall Street Journal, August 25, 2016.[31]

This system has continued because of two directives CEOs have long given HR: Keep people happy and don't get us sued.

This may have made sense when health care benefits were a small percentage of the company's budget, but decades of hyper-inflating costs have made it the second or third largest expense. Also, it's hard to make the argument that a company is keeping employees happy when health insurance has the lowest customer satisfaction of any industry and high-deductible plans have suddenly become the norm.

I'm regularly asked to speak to benefits consultants, business coalitions, nonprofit associations, and public-sector organizations about how to tackle this situation. The overriding sentiment I find is that organization executives and benefits leaders have reached their breaking point financially and are no longer willing to accept that every year they're obligated to get less and pay more for health benefits. More than anything else, the recognition that their decisions have contributed to the worsening of the opioid crisis is a wake-up call.

David Contorno is a leading benefits consultant who contributed to Chapter 12. One of the reasons he's completely transformed his approach has been the impact he's seen in his client base. In the last year, 22 people on the health plans of his clients died of opioid overdoses. All but two were dependents aged 17-25. There may be nothing more painful than losing a child. These tragedies are part of the reason he's become so passionate about advocating for Direct Primary Care, since undermining this primary care model has been so pervasive and has created fertile ground for overprescribing opioids.

A Breach of Fiduciary Responsibility

If health care is the immediate cause of the economic depression of middle-class workers, the underlying cause is a breach of fiduciary duty by their employers. While there is a lot of attention paid to the Obamacare exchanges, they only represent about seven percent of the population. Understandably, Medicare and Medicaid get a lot of attention, but the fact is that employers collectively pick up the biggest portion of the health care tab and non-retirees overwhelmingly get their health insurance through the workplace. ERISA, which regulates both health and retirement plans, requires employers to act in their employees' interest in providing these benefits. While employers are very good at doing this with retirement plans, they are seriously bad at doing this with health plans.

Could a simple rule clarification trigger a correction of the whole system?

From where I sit, it seems that all the Department of Labor (DOL) needs to do is state that *health benefits dollars are considered the employees' money*—not the employer's. That is, spending on health benefits should be held to the same fiduciary standards as retirement benefits, as the DOL states on their website. (https://www.dol.gov/general/topic/health-plans/fiduciaryresp). That would mean the widespread lack of transparency on fees and conflicts of interest would become a thing of the past.

Sean Schantzen, a former practicing securities attorney who is relatively new to health care, has pointed out that someone in financial services would land in jail or in civil court for breach of fiduciary duty for following what is standard operating procedure in health care. For example, in the class action suit brought by employees against Edison International, the petitioners alleged that Edison breached its fiduciary duties by offering participants in the 401(k) plan retail share classes of mutual funds when lower-priced institutional share classes were available. The employees won a unanimous verdict at the U.S. Supreme Court. By comparison, benefits brokers receive cash bonuses for keeping 90 percent of their clients in disadvantageous arrangements with specific insurers.

In fairness to the Department of Labor, prior to high-deductible plans, it was once easier to argue that health benefits spending was the "employer's money." But today, 51 percent of the workforce has a deductible of more than $1,000. With cost sharing and high deductibles, employees are typically paying approximately 30 percent of health benefits costs.

The Health Rosetta

I believe the Health Rosetta is the way forward. The Health Rosetta is an ever-evolving collection of principles and best practices that I and many like-minded professional colleagues have put together that's a blueprint for sustainably reducing costs and improving care. It's built on real-life successes, not theory. It simplifies the path for you to achieve similar results.

In the old model of health care, the supply side dictated the pricing and terms. Today, forward-looking organizations refuse to leave these areas unmanaged. The wisest are turning health care costs, which many view as a liability, into a source of competitive advantage. They have found they can reduce spending by 20 percent or more per capita while providing better benefits than 99 percent of the workforce. In other words, the best way to slash health care costs is to *improve* the quality of those benefits. The Health Rosetta makes it easier to follow these leaders.

The Health Rosetta mission is to accelerate adoption of these proven approaches. It focuses on practical, non-partisan fixes to how we pay for care, what we buy, and how we manage benefits. It helps public and private employers and unions reduce health benefits costs while providing better care for the 150 million Americans who receive health benefits through their jobs.

While this book focuses on non-government-paid health care, the biggest missed opportunity may be at the state and federal level. The public sector is a large employer itself, representing a broad cross-section of society. Public sector employers have all the same opportunities as private sector employers to greatly improve the value they receive.

Broadly speaking, the two biggest problems in the U.S. health care system are pricing failure (no correlation between price and health outcomes) and overtreatment. These problems are pervasive in both publicly and privately funded health care benefits. Policy makers would be wise to test and prove their models of reform with the public-sector workforce. Fortunately, they have widespread examples of success to follow. The Health Rosetta aggregates these into an understandable blueprint.

Here are a few of the Health Rosetta's foundational components:

- **Transparent Advisor Relationships.** All direct and indirect revenue sources benefits that advisors receive are disclosed to their clients.
- **Active ERISA plan management.** Employers deeply manage budgets in every other area of spending. Why not health benefits? Internal fiduciary oversight is critical.
- **Value-based primary care.** Properly conceptualized and incentivized primary care is the front line of defense against downstream costs.
- **Concierge services.** Navigating health care is complex, even for those of us in the industry. Employees need access to trusted, aligned resources.
- **Transparent open networks.** Cost and quality are often inversely correlated in health care. Focusing on better quality and outcomes is the path to lower costs. This is particularly true for addressing high-cost outlier claims that make up the majority of spending.
- **Payment integrity.** Ensuring claims are paid correctly and tackling fraud is a critical step to high-performance benefits.
- **Transparent pharmacy benefits.** Purchasers need true transparency of data to control decision making.

So, if fixes already exist, why isn't everyone using them?

Health care's redemption is a classic example of solutions hidden in plain sight. Remember the movies *The Big Short* and *Moneyball*? As noted business consultant Ric Merrifield, author of *Rethink: A Business Manifesto for Cutting Costs and Boosting Innovation,* has pointed out, their shared theme was that in the face of a mountain of evidence that corrupt practices were destroying people's lives and savings (not to mention the housing market), no one paid attention: Wall Street and federal regulators didn't downgrade the credit ratings of mortgage backed securities even when the mountain was right in front of them.

Health care is in the same place the banking industry was in the early 2000s. My hope is that this book will contribute to a health care turnaround even more profound and longer lasting than that of banking.

Key Take-aways

- Despite almost no changes to the underlying costs of health care, there's an annual ritual designed to create the perception that costs have increased. Although it is inaccurate, the misperception is widely believed to be true.
- The opioid crisis has amplified the awakening of benefits professionals that they have unwittingly enabled the opioid crisis by the health plans they've deployed.
- Forward-looking industry leaders have created and proven wise health care purchasing and delivery that serves as a model for the next 50 years of health care.

CHAPTER 3

AMERICA HAS GONE TO WAR FOR FAR LESS

"Health is worth more than learning." – Thomas Jefferson

One definition of an economic depression is two or more years of income decline. Since the middle class has seen wages decline over the last 20 years after adjusting for inflation (see Figure 2), they have been experiencing a depression for nearly twenty years. Here's why.

Employers spend more on payroll than ever, yet virtually the entire increase has gone to health care costs, as Rand concluded in their report, *How Does Growth in Health Care Costs Affect the American Family?*[32] In many cases, those costs have literally taken all of the payroll increases for middle class employees. In Mobile, Alabama last year, the Public Education Employees Health Insurance Plan board voted to raise health care insurance premiums for families from $177/month to $307/month. This promptly ate up the state-approved 4 percent pay raise for employees that make less than $75,000 a year.[33] Both employees and employers (public and private) bear the burden of these huge premium increases.

Accurate Box Co. CEO Lisa Hirsh said that 25 years ago health care benefits were five percent of an employee's total compensation at her company. Today, that cost can be 30, 40, or even

50 percent of total compensation. "When family health care costs are $30,000 a year and the person is making $30,000, their total package could be $60,000, but they're not seeing it."[34]

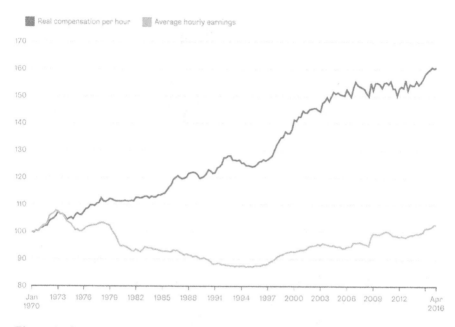

Figure 2. Compensation, including Benefits, versus Take-Home Pay. Includes bene-fits, indexed to 100, and adjusted for inflation. Source: Barry Ritholtz, "Health Care Costs Ate Your Pay Raises."[35]

A Sneak Attack

Imagine if a foreign country were causing this kind of collateral damage on our economy. We'd go to war in a second. Yet, we haven't. Evidence of the industry's "sneak attack" on the U.S. is clear. To wit...

The greatest public health crisis in 100 years is a crisis created entirely by health care industry dysfunction

As we saw in Chapter 1, the opioid crisis is a predictable outcome of a profoundly broken health care system. Every two weeks, as many people as died on 9/11 die from overdoses— and overdoses are underreported due to stigma. Last year, more people died of opioid overdoses than Americans killed during the Vietnam War.[36] The vast majority of opioid use disorders begin with a patient following doctor's orders. Many high-function individuals are able to hide their addiction from their friends and co-workers. For example, Kristin Labott's nurse colleagues didn't find out until she was cuffed and taken away to jail;[37] fortunately, she has been in recovery for over a decade. However, while I was writing Chapter 1, a leader in the public health department of one of the biggest cities in America died of an opioid overdose. Her friends knew the cause of death, but her husband wanted it reported as a heart attack to protect her reputation or perhaps a life insurance policy that limits payouts related to drug-related deaths.

Household income has been devastated by health care costs.

According to an article in the *Annals of Family Medicine*, from 2000 to 2009, the average annual increase in insurance premiums was eight percent. During the same timeframe, household incomes rose an average of 2.1 percent. If health insurance premiums and national wages continue to grow at these rates, the average cost of a family health insurance premium will equal 50 percent of its household income by 2021—and exceed 100 percent of household income by 2033.[38] This is at least partly to blame for the fact that nearly seven in 10 Americans have less than $1,000 in savings.[39]

Illness or medical bills are a major contributor to bankruptcies

In 2013, more than 1.5 million Americans lived in households that experienced a health-related bankruptcy. More than three-quarters of those people had insurance.[40] Some say medical bills may also be the top cause of homelessness. Nearly half of all GoFundMe crowdfunding campaigns are to pay for medical-related expenses.[41]

State-level data demonstrate that health care is choking other budgets such as education.

Massachusetts is a cautionary tale. Its move to almost universal health care insurance in 2006 became the model for reform nationwide, the Affordable Care Act. While the state did see coverage increases, Figure 3 shows this came at a 37 percent increase in health care costs. As a result, funding in education decreased by 12.2 percent, mental health by 22.2 percent, and local aid by 50.5 percent. Frequently, in education, what used to be paid for by taxes has been cut entirely and parents or teachers have to raise money to ensure their children get core school programs. In other words, we're stealing our kids' future.

Massachusetts was also forced to cut infrastructure spending, which dropped 14 percent. And Massachusetts is hardly alone. At the local, state, and federal level, drinking water has become unsafe, trains are literally going off the tracks, and bridges are falling into rivers as health care costs have starved budgets of infrastructure investment.

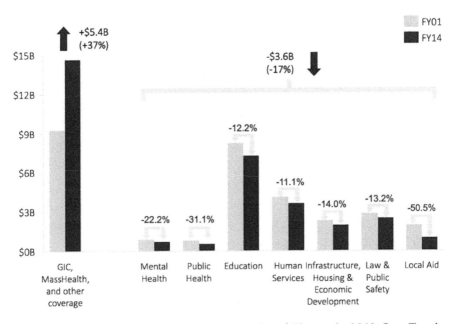

Figure 3. Source: Health Policy Commission, "List of Figures in 2013 Cost Trends Report by the Health Policy Commission."[42]

Between 2004 and 2014, officials in the little town of China, Maine, saw health insurance costs go up 141 percent to $200,000 per year for 11 municipal employees; the cost for just one of those employees with dependents equals the town's entire parks and recreation budget or the operating budget for one of its three volunteer fire departments. Instead of repaving roads, China is patching budgets. Beyond these microcosms, there are hundreds of millions of dollars in unfunded pension commitments around the country.[43]

More than 210,000 people die each year from preventable medical error in hospitals and other health care settings.[44]

It's the fifth leading cause of death in the U.S. after respiratory disease, accidents, stroke, and Alzheimer's.[45] Note that this is approaches the number of soldiers killed in combat during WWII.[46]

These deaths are primarily due to infections, along with errors in prescribing and administering drugs, mistaken diagnoses, botched surgeries and procedures, falls, and communication lapses from one care provider to another. The number of preventable adverse events associated with hospital care every day is 10,000—the medical equivalent of "friendly fire" happening seven times per minute. As with most cases of friendly fire, it's leadership and design that are most often at fault, rather than individuals. For detailed information on this subject, check out Sarah Kliff's powerful exposé on the flawed medical culture, "Do No Harm,"[47] and Dr. Marty Makary's book, *Unaccountable*,[48] which bring these statistics to life in devastating detail.

Hyperinflating health care costs have significantly reduced retirement savings.

I did some very rough, back-of-envelope calculations on what could be put into people's retirement plans if not for hyperinflating health care costs. I used historical rates of inflation, S&P growth, and health care premiums. Over 30 years, the average American household would have around $1,000,000 in their retirement account (assuming growth in an S&P index fund).[49] As things stand, the majority of Americans have next to no retirement savings and 68 percent of millennials aren't participating in a job-related retirement plan.[50]

There are unprecedented levels of dissatisfaction and burnout by doctors.

According to a Doctors Company survey of 5,000 physicians, nine out of 10 physician respondents indicated an unwillingness to recommend health care as a profession.[51] A major reason is the layering of more and more bureaucracy. A recent study found that for every hour physicians see patients, they spend nearly two additional hours on recordkeeping.[52] Another reason is that they're forced to see too many patients too fast, robbing them and patients of the ability to effectively diagnose or of any sense of connection or satisfaction.[53] Sadly, doctors have the highest rate of suicide of any profession.[54]

The High Cost of Poor Care

Dying or end-of-life care is a good example of how we over-spend on care we shouldn't be receiving in the first place. As renowned physician, policy analyst, and author Atul Gawande covered in his book *Being Mortal: Medicine and What Matters in the End*, the U.S. does a horrendous job dealing with end-of-life issues. This often leads, as Ken Murray, MD put it, to "misery we would not inflict on a terrorist" for our loved ones.[55] It also squanders billions of dollars. Approximately 30 percent of all Medicare spending is in the last six months of life, most of it unnecessary and much of it harmful.

Knowing the limits of medicine and what impacts quality of life, many doctors die differently than the rest of us, said Murray, meaning they die with much less intervention (and cost). People in La Crosse, Wisconsin, happily for them, are also not like the rest of us: 96 percent of residents have advance directives saying how they wish to be treated at the end of life—and those wishes are respected. Now look at the cost differential: $18,000 for care in the last two years of life in La Crosse vs. a national average of $26,000. At one hospital in New York City, this is more than $75,000.[56]

Musculoskeletal (MSK) procedures, primarily surgeries such as knee replacements and spinal fusions, are another example of our overspending on care we don't want or need. These unnecessary MSK procedures are one of the significant on-ramps to opioid use disorders. The *Atlantic* reported in "When Evidence Says No, but Doctors Say Yes" how pervasive overtreatment is in areas such as stents and musculoskeletal procedures.[57] In fact, benefits expert Brian Klepper, formerly CEO of the National Alliance of Health Care Purchaser Coalitions, estimates that two percent of the entire U.S. economy (not just health care) is wasted on non-evidence-based MSK procedures that add no value. How can that be? Health care spending is nearly 20 percent of the national economy,

MSK procedures are typically 20 percent of health care spending, and only 50 percent of MSK procedures are evidence-based.[58]

Health care is a three-trillion-dollar industry and 30 cents of every one of those dollars spent on health care is wasted, according to the Institute of Medicine. In 2009, that was $750 billion. Imagine what we could do with that money:[59]

- Send every 17- and 18-year-old to a state university for four years
- Fund the Department of Defense for a year
- Cover all hospital and medical care for veterans for 51 years
- Pay for all U.S. economic aid to foreign countries for 36 years (and still have $14 billion left over)
- Cover all annual health care costs for the uninsured six times over

Yet, despite all this waste and devastation, and despite employers spending huge sums to keep up with hyperinflating costs, the reality is that status quo health benefits are a horrible value proposition for employers and individuals.

For example, flawed reimbursement incentives have made primary care a "loss leader," like milk in the back of the grocery store (i.e., a low-margin item designed to get customers to purchase high margin items). The result is rushed appointments, unnecessary referrals to specialty care, over-prescribing, and lower pay, making the discipline increasingly unappealing to physicians. Unsurprisingly, this has led to a primary care shortage. This leads to long wait times to see a primary care physician or no access at all, which can cause small health care fires to become 5-alarm medical infernos. In short, undervaluing primary care is the root cause of medically unnecessary office appointments, clogged waiting rooms, and unconscionable delays in care for people who truly need a face-to-face encounter.

Not surprisingly, Figure 4 shows that Net Promoter Scores, a common measure of customer satisfaction, shows the health insurance industry is lower than even cable companies.

Health Insurance: Lowest Customer Satisfaction of Any Industry

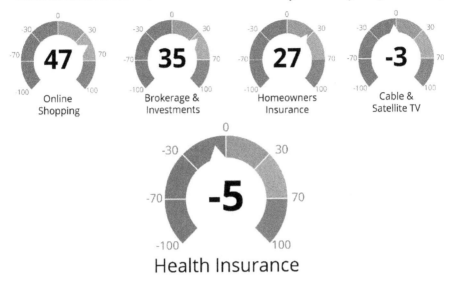

Figure 4. Note that some industries have so many detractors that the score becomes negative.[60]

A Way Out

While the status quo "preservatives" squabble in DC, forward-leaning individuals and organizations aren't waiting around. They see the threat for what it is and are creating examples for all of us to follow. There is a budding partnership between clinicians dissatisfied with the status quo, citizens who realize they have more power than they'd imagined, and communities no longer willing to passively accept further theft of the American dream.

Jeffrey Brenner, MD—executive director of The Camden Coalition of Health Care Providers and MacArthur Genius Award winner for his work using data to identify and improve the care of high-cost, high-need patients—put it succinctly in a *Freakonomics* interview: "There comes a point in a democracy when the public's had enough and they stand up."[61] For many across all segments of health care and all political persuasions, that time is now.

The three most trusted professions in the U.S. are nurses, doctors, and pharmacists. A key reason I love working in the health care industry is the great people I've gotten to know. However, great people inside a flawed system will always underperform those in a great system.

While it will take people of all stripes to lead the movement, doctors have a unique role to play. In fact, some doctors are leading the revolution. Here are just two examples.

Rushika Fernandopulle, MD

Fernandopulle is a practicing physician and cofounder and CEO of Iora Health, a health care services firm based in Boston. He was also the first executive director of the Harvard Interfaculty Program for Health Systems Improvement and managing director of the Clinical Initiatives Center at the Advisory Board Company. Fernandopulle was among the first to understand that caring for the care team is foundational to achieving the best outcomes and reducing unnecessary costs and treatment. His work was featured in *The New Yorker* article "Hot Spotters," which highlighted the best ways to care for the sickest patients in our cities.[62]

Iora's mission is to build a radically new primary care model that improves quality and service, while reducing overall costs. It has opened successful practices in a wide variety of clinic settings, serving casino union workers, university employees, freelancers, undocumented workers, and Medicare recipients.

Full disclosure: My parents are in a Medicare Advantage program that has Iora Health as a key primary care partner.

Dr. Mark Tomasulo, D.O.

With an ever-changing health care system and frustration among both doctors and patients, Tomasulo founded PeakMed Primary Care with a goal of redefining access and decreasing health care costs. He realized that the business of health care has rapidly changed over the last 15 years and, as a result, the doctor-patient relationship has suffered. Doctors are reluctant to enter the specialty of Family Medicine and senior mentoring physicians are retiring early.

The restructuring of the health care system has increased costs to the patient as well as to the employer, creating a barrier to true health care. PeakMed's disruptive approach in health care has created a platform allowing doctors and patients to communicate, manage, and collaborate individualized care plans without the constraints of a broken system. PeakMed has grown into one of the most successful Direct Primary Care organizations through their success working directly for individual patients as well as individuals sponsored by their employer.

Tomasulo currently holds the title of Chief Medical Officer where he focuses on disruptive innovation and bending the curve of cost and access in health care. Tomasulo completed his medical training through the United States Army. He served eight years in the Army as one of the top officers in his field and was part of small unit deployments in support of Operation Iraqi Freedom.

For health care revolutionaries, it's what Ronald Reagan called Morning in America.

Key Take-aways

- The health care system itself has become the greatest immediate threat to our freedom to pursue health and the American Dream. The opioid crisis serves as a wake-up call to the even broader crisis in health care.
- Health care has redistributed virtually all employer increased spending from employees to an under-performing health care system over the last 20 years creating an economic depression for the working and middle class.
- Health care is choking funding for education, public infrastructure, and social services.
- Despite spending far more than any country in the world, there are 10,000 instances per day of preventable medical mistakes, causing unnecessary suffering and spending.
- Physician leaders are proving there are ways to get twice the health care at half the cost.

Rosie the Restorer

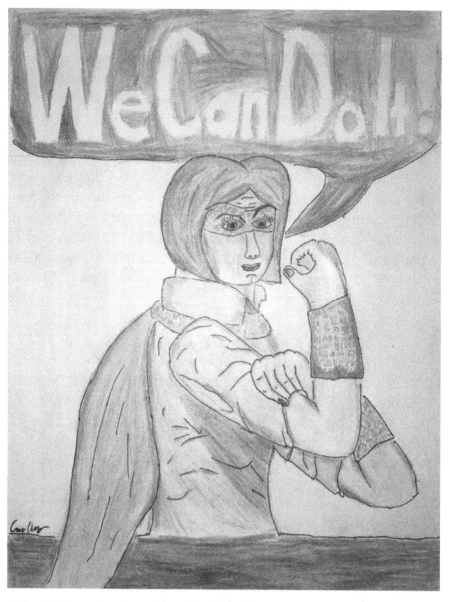

In family discussions about the need to fix health care, I explained to my son how every now and then the country is able to really pull together. I used Rosie the Riveter as a symbol from WWII. We decided we needed a new symbol of someone who was truly heroic and could get the job—any job—done. My son knew instantly who it should be: mom! Rosie the Restorer here is a mashup of a superhero, a mom, and Rosie the Riveter. [Courtesy of Cameron Chase, age 12]

PITTSBURGH (ALLEGHENY COUNTY) SCHOOLS

Investing in Kids While Ensuring Teachers Receive Better Care

Bucking old habits that are devastating education funding elsewhere, forward-looking teacher union and school board leaders in Allegheny County, Pennsylvania are proving that it's not really so difficult to slay the health care cost beast and save their kids' future—even in an expensive and contentious health care market. Understandably, unions want their members to be compensated fairly and keep schools from being decimated. Recognizing that they share the same goals, the school board decided to take a new approach.

Assuming the current trend continues, kindergartners entering Pittsburgh area schools will collectively have $2 billion more available to invest in education and services over the course of their school years than their counterparts across the state in Philadelphia. In Philadelphia, schools pay $8,815 per member for teacher health benefits. The Allegheny County Schools Health Insurance Consortium (ACSHIC), with 48,000 covered lives, pays $4,661 per member—$199 million less per year. Class sizes in Pittsburgh are 30 percent smaller, teachers are paid better with better benefits, and there are four times as many librarians.

Rewarding Wise Decisions

Jan Klein, ACSHIC's business manager, describes a model that is very consistent with the Health Rosetta blueprint. In a nutshell, they make smart decisions free or nearly free (e.g., primary care is free, and going to high-quality care providers involves very low or no copays or deductibles) and poor decisions expensive (e.g., pay more to see higher cost, lower quality care providers). It's a much more subtle, yet more effective, strategy than blunt-instrument, high-deductible plans that often lead to deferred care, bankruptcies, reduced teacher compensation, fewer arts programs… the list goes on.

The consortium is managed by 24 trustees, equal parts labor and management. When consultants attend consortium meetings, they often can't tell who is who. Many times, union leaders are more aggressive in pushing forward new initiatives. While other employers have blithely accepted five to 20 percent annual health care cost increases, the consortium spent $233 million in annual claims in 2016—*down* from $241 million in 2014. The consortium is able to manage their costs without any stop loss insurance because they have control over what they call their benefit grid, a program that was defined and embraced by both union leaders and teachers.

They've accomplished this, even though care provider organization consolidation in Western Pennsylvania has reduced competition and raised health care costs with little to no improvement in quality of care—and despite an ongoing war between the largest hospital, the University of Pittsburgh Medical Center (UPMC), and the largest local insurance carrier, Highmark.

Understanding that the best way to spend less is to improve health care quality, ACSHIC found that the path began with the following steps:

- Educating consortium trustees on quality rankings of hospitals, including sending them to a Pittsburgh Business Group on Health forum
- Retrieving hospital quality data through third-party data and tools (e.g., Imagine Health, CareChex, and Innovu)
- Validating vendor information by confirming it was not influenced by bias
- Selecting the most effective resources by identifying credible partners/vendors

Once educated, the trustees provided the following direction to the team developing the new school district health plan.

- Use quality measures from respected third-party sources.
- Create tiered products so people are free to go wherever they want for care—but they pay more if they choose sites that have lower quality and value.
- Focus on ease of access to regional clinics and hospitals.
- Focus on the relationship between cost and quality (the former turned out not to be indicative of the latter).
- Educate members, especially about why the local academic medical center was placed in a high-cost tier (it wasn't the highest-quality facility for many kinds of care).
- Address member concerns (e.g., will this really save money?) through continuous communication.

Results

Health care purchasing before (October 2013 - September 2014)

# 1 Hospital in the region (highest quality rating)	#23 Hospital in the region (low quality rating)
33,352 Services*	31,047 Services
293 Admits	362 Admits
$4,941,146 in total costs	$15,089,972 in total costs

*Services include imaging, lab test, outpatient procedures, etc.

Intervention to improve value: tiered benefit offerings

- The enhanced tier has NO deductible and pays 100% of hospital charges.
- The standard tier has a deductible and pays 80% of hospital charges.
- Out-of-network care has a larger deductible and pays 50% of hospital charges.
- Lower cost and higher quality is determined by third-party, independent benchmarks.

Health care purchasing after (October 2015 - September 2016)

#1 Hospital in the region (highest quality rating)	#23 Hospital in the region (low quality rating!)
40,046 Services (up 20%)	6,620 Services (down 79%)
328 Admits (up 12%)	113 Admits (down 69%)
$7,170,357 in total costs (up 45%)	$5,548,832 in total costs (down 63%)

In sum, the consortium reduced hospital spending by

$7.36 million, a 36.8% reduction

*Services include imaging, lab test, outpatient procedures, etc.

Going Forward

The consortium expects to continue enhancing benefits with only a very modest premium increase of 1.9 percent for members. Here are a few plan attributes going forward.

- The enhanced tier has no deductibles.
- Primary care visits have no copay.
- Specialist visits have a $10 copay.
- An employee assistance program provider.
- A second opinion service.

Their determination to serve kids led education leaders in Pittsburgh to move past tired assumptions about labor and management being forever at odds over health benefits. With any luck, their steely resolve in the face of local challenges will inspire teachers' unions and school boards throughout the country to say NO to health care stealing our kids' future. Imagine how much better schools would be if every school district replicated Pittsburgh's approach. If you are a parent or community member, share (www.healthrosetta.org/schools) with leaders in your local schools for this and other examples of success. You can find calculators on how avoiding wasted health care bureaucracy can allow for health and well-being in our future and kids.

CHAPTER 4

HEALTH CARE COSTS ARE FLAT DESPITE WHAT YOU HAVE HEARD

Jeanne Pinder

"If it wasn't complicated, it wouldn't be allowed to happen. The complexity disguises what is happening. If it's so complicated you can't understand it, then you can't question it." – Michael Lewis

A curious thing has happened in health care pricing in this country. While insurance premiums and prices for common procedures for insured people go up and up and up, cash or negotiated self-pay prices* for many procedures vary little from year to year.

But wait, I can hear you saying, health care prices always go up, don't they? They do if they go through a PPO or major insurance carrier. But for the most part, negotiated cash or self- pay prices don't, at least not consistently. Sometimes, they modestly increase, but more often, they stay the same—or even go down from year to year. Our team of journalists noticed this pattern when we began comparing data sets year over year from the same locations.

---

* For the purposes of this book, a "cash price" is what a provider charges an individual who is either paying directly, using a check or credit card, or is covered by an employer or union that pays immediately under a direct contract that bypasses the insurance claims processing process.

We have been surveying care providers about their cash or self-pay prices for five years and have a very good set of data for 13 metro areas. Some did, indeed, raise rates regularly, but they tended to be the higher-priced care providers in the first place. Overall, the flatline pattern is clear.

For example, we recently re-reported our New York City cash prices. The following figures show the trend for MRIs and ultrasounds. Note the wild variation in pricing among care providers, which persists across regions, cities, and even within individual health care systems and hospitals. This reflects yet another health care cost problem: unpredictability and variability of cost for the same procedures. *

---

* It's worth noting that overall hyperinflation in health care spending is multivariate. It comes partially from the issues discussed here. Another major source is care and procedures that shouldn't happen at all, as a result of overuse, misdiagnosis, unnecessary, or ineffective treatment and procedures. We discuss this separate but related issue in Chapter 12.

Procedure: Pelvic Ultrasound

Facility	Code	2011	2012	2013	2017
Dynamic Medical Imaging	76856	X	$125	$125	$125
Neighborhood Radiology	76856	X	X	$150	$132
New Millennium Medical	76856	X	$150	$150	$150
Hudson Valley Radiological Associates	76856	$198	$198	$213	$158
Rochester General Hospital	76856	X	X	$229	$212
Greenwich Radiology Group	76856	X	X	$344	$344
Brooklyn Heights Imaging	76856	X	$185	$185	$375
Highway Imaging Associates	76856	X	$175	$175	$375
Diagnostic Imaging of Millford	76856	X	X	$314	$413
East River Medical Imaging	76856	X	$377	$377	$754
Lawrence Hospital	76856	X	X	$654	$792
Crescent Radiology	76856	$150	$150	X	X
Diagnostic Imaging Services Bronxville	76856	$469	$491	X	X
Empire Imaging	76856	$175	$200	X	X
Manhasset Diagnostic	76856	$300	$85	X	X
New York Imagery	76856	$350	$207	X	X
New York Westchester Square Med. Center	76856	$648	$700	X	X
Park Avenue Radiologists	76856	$366	$325	X	X

Procedure: Lower back MRI without contrast

Facility	Code	2011	2012	2013	2017
Advanced Radiology	72148	$1,160	$1,160	$1,093	$0
Queens Radiology/Olympic Open MRI	72148	$400	$450	$450	$0
Neighborhood Radiology	72148	X	$150	$150	$150
Radiology of Westchester	72148	X	X	$450	$450
Middle Village Radiology	72148	$350	$450	$450	$500
New Rochelle Radiology	72148	X	X	$500	$500
Greater Waterbury Imaging Center	72148	X	$185	$185	$375
Housatonic Valley Radiology Assoc.	72148	X	X	$816	$627
East River Medical Imaging	72148	$1,900	$1,900	$1,200	$1,900
Columbus Circle Imaging	72148	X	X	$1,200	$2,600
East Manhattan Diagnostic Imaging	72148	X	X	$1,200	$2,600
Union Square Diagnostic Imaging	72148	$800	$1,800	$1,200	$2,600
Advanced Radiology	72148	$1,064	$556	X	X
Astoria Medical Imaging	72148	$450	$1,200	X	X
Park Avenue Radiologists	72148	$1,000	$0	X	X

Source: ClearHealthCosts. Used with Permission.[63]

Unpredictable Costs

Premiums go up, deductibles go up, out-of-pocket spending goes up, as Figure 5 shows. Inexorably, inevitably. Or so we are told. But if you look deeper, pricing and costs are completely unpredictable.

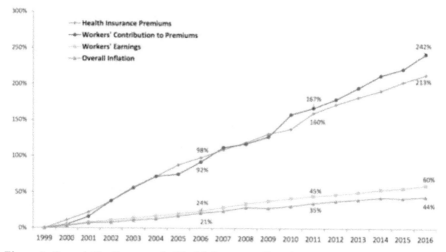

Figure 5. Cumulative Increases in Health Insurance Premiums, General Annual Deductibles, Inflation, and Workers' Earnings, 2011-2016. Source: Employer Health Benefit Survey 2016, Kaiser Family Foundation and Health Research & Education Trust.[64]

Below is a sample of comparative prices graciously given to us a couple of years ago by a care provider organization. The table below shows charged rates, reimbursement rates, and individual responsibility for a selected group of procedures at the organization. Each row is for a different individual on a different health plan. As you can see, if you have a $10,000 deductible, you might exhaust that deductible before you get to anything else, depending on the "insurance paid" or "negotiated" rate. Or, you might spend only $2,681 toward your deductible.

Example 1: Knee arthroscopy

Charges range from $13,452 to $19,187.
Insurance payments range from $2,681 to $13,607,
a *508% variation in the actual paid amount*

CPTCode	Billed, Cash or Self-Pay Price	Insurance Paid Amt.	Patient Responsibility
29881	$15,233.58	$2,681.36	$350
29881	$19,187.85	$3,795.20	$948.80
29881	$13,452.86	$9,080.77	$1,008.91
29881	$18,142.68	$13,607	$0

Example 2: Repair Initial inguinal hernia (No. 1 and No. 2)

Charges range from $13,950 to $22,184.
Payments range from $2,515 to $12,281,
a *500% variation in the actual paid amount*

Figure #1

CPT Code	Billed, Cash or Self-Pay Price	Insurance Paid Amt.	Patient Responsibility
36561	$13,950.29	$2,514.75	$641.52
36561	$15,680.49	$8,467.46	$940.83
36561	$15,948.16	$11,961.10	$0

Figure #2

CPT Code	Billed, Cash or Self-Pay Price	Insurance Paid Amt.	Patient Responsibility
49505	$22,183.85	$3,008.58	$767.50
49505	$17,011.54	$4,576	$1,144
49505	$18,193.78	$12,280.80	$1,364.53

Example 3: Carpal tunnel surgery

Charges range from $9,694 to $11,721.
Payments range from $1,953 to $7,079,
a *362% variation in the actual paid amount*

CPT Code	Billed, Cash or Self-Pay Price	Insurance Paid Amt.	Patient Responsibility
64721	$9,694.24	$1,953.47	$0
64721	$11,106.59	$3,174.30	$452.70
64721	$11,721.45	$3,501	$0
64721	$10,097.93	$7,079.25	$494.20

Example 4: Cataract surgery with intraocular lens (IOL)

Charges from $10,456 to $12,831.
Insurance payments range from $2,474 to $8,024,
a *324% variation in the actual paid amount*

CPT Code	Billed, Cash or Self-Pay Price	Insurance Paid Amt.	Patient Responsibility
66984	$10,456.39	$2,473.63	$0
66984	$12,831.26	$2,473.63	$0
66984	$10,878.50	$2,473.63	$0
66984	$10,606.54	$4,328	$100
66984	$11,503.16	$8,024.07	$603.30

Source: ClearHealthCosts. Used with permission.[65]

If you're not surprised and shocked yet, get ready. Insured individuals who ask for cash prices pay less than other insured individuals. For example, in San Francisco, Castro Valley Open MRI charges $475 cash for a lower back MRI. An insured individual who asked for a cash price for the same MRI at a different care provider knocked a $1,850 bill down to $580. A different insured individual was initially charged $5,667 for the same MRI at a third care provider. Their insurer paid $2,367, and the individual was asked to pay $1,114.54, a total of $3,471.54 to the third care provider for the same $475 MRI. It's enough to make your head spin.

However, there's a trend toward transparency for competitive and regulatory reasons. For example, Surgery Center of Oklahoma founder, Keith Smith, MD, has been publicizing cash prices online for nearly nine years.

"I've only changed them four times," he said. "And in every case, I lowered them. So, I think I could make a compelling case that prices are actually falling."

Smith is still making money too, he said, often paying doctors more for procedures than insurers. "If we realize some efficiency in our practice that we've not seen before, then our inclination is to pass that savings along to the buyer and make ourselves even more competitive in the market."

More and more providers are following his practice of posting cash prices publicly, pushing us closer to the day when anyone can walk into a facility or physician's office with a price and insist they step up and match it.

Third Parties, Intermediaries, and Escalator Clauses

So, what causes insurance premiums and noncash prices to continue going up? For one thing, contracts between providers and carriers can include things like automatic escalator clauses, which stipulate that payment rates automatically increase each year.

Then there's the chargemaster, the list of prices at a hospital or other health care provider. Here's how one hospital executive explained the chargemaster to me: "Bob in accounting made that list in the 1960s, and we just raise prices every year. But don't tell anybody—we like them to think it's because our cost of business keeps going up, and because of uncompensated care, and because of the burden of keeping an ER open 24-7, and because health care is just expensive."

And then there are all the people behind the scenes between you and your doctor, each taking a dime or a dollar or a hundred dollars out of every transaction. For example, a good size hospital probably has multiple vice presidents for strategic planning, armies of business-office workers, pricing consultants, and people to make revenue-cycle management projections—just as the insurance company does.

"There are a lot of people in corporate medicine who make a ton of money off the lack of market-competitive pricing," Smith said. "And these people don't want to give that game up." But Smith says it's a myth that insurance companies care about prices. "They really don't. All they care about are charges because they're in the business of selling discounts. The higher the prices are to start with, the more money they make in discounting those prices. So that's part of the problem; a PPO will say that their discount saved an employer tens of thousands of dollars—in which they naturally share."

Turning Things Around

Joining Smith in his cynicism is Mike Dendy, who predicts the PPO concept will die out over the next few years.

Dendy was the CEO of Advanced Medical Pricing Solutions, a Georgia-based company that does health cost management for self-insured employer health plans. They help employers beat back costs using tools like close scrutiny of bills, the formation of narrower networks, direct contracting between providers and employers, and reference-based pricing services, often based on Medicare reimbursement rates. Dendy said providers commonly charge 300 to 500 percent of Medicare's rate and even the largest employers pay 250 percent on average, including both in and out-of-network claims, although he's seen hospitals creep up to 700 percent.

"The last report I saw showed the average spending by an employer group last year was about $18,300 per employee," he said. "It's getting unsustainable—and every 4 or 5 percent increase now is a lot bigger than it was 20 years ago. The situation can be remedied, but you need consumerism to make it happen: incentives or disincentives for the consumer. And then you need technology and information immediately available, so people can make the correct decision in non-emergency situations."

Dendy further predicted that the insurance market will move toward defined contribution plans, where an employer's spending would be limited in scope. He compared employer health policies with travel policies. If you're traveling for the company, he said, the company limits your outlay.

"Nobody thinks they're being grossly burdened by not being able to stay at the Four Seasons and eat steak five times a day (unless they're paying for it themselves). But under current health insurance arrangements, via a PPO, an employee is free to choose an expensive MRI or an expensive hospital—and that raises everybody's premiums," he said.

Jeanne Pinder is founder and CEO of ClearHealthCosts, an independent health care research organization; its team of independent journalists is dedicated to finding and publishing costs for medical procedures and items.

Key Take-aways

- Prices are flat in the real market – the direct pay and cash-based market – for the vast majority of health care costs.
- Costs haven't changed for most inputs into health care. Prices aren't correlated with underlying costs.
- Escalator and gag clauses create an opaque market where hospitals and insurance companies have a shared objective for prices to go up irrespective of costs.

CHAPTER 5

WHAT YOU DON'T KNOW ABOUT THE PRESSURES AND CONSTRAINTS FACING INSURANCE EXECUTIVES COSTS YOU DEARLY

"What You Don't Know Will Hurt You. Ignorance is Not Bliss."–
Jim Rohn

For all the recent talk about accountable care organizations, there is a distinct lack of accountability when it comes to health care costs. Hospitals blame insurance companies, insurance companies blame hospitals, providers blame the government, and everyone blames drug companies. Even though many organizations have woken up to the fact that they can get better bang for their buck if they are self-insured, most self-insured organizations still don't pay close attention to the critical details that often have the most dramatic impact on their bottom line.

Here's why: Virtually every conversation I have with employers reveals a profound lack of understanding of market dynamics, constraints, and incentives that health insurance company executives face. For the most part, these executives are good people operating perfectly rationally, given the drivers and constraints of their business. These constraints include care provider organization practices, Wall Street profit expectations, employer/ employee demands (yes, you!), and regulatory issues. Unfortunately, the net result incentivizes redistributing profits from you and your community to the health care industry. In short, their incentives are not aligned with yours. Like hospitals (the biggest recipient of your health care dollars), insurance companies win when health care costs go up.

Understanding the specific pressures facing insurance company executives will help you more effectively negotiate and drive better value from your health dollars. Plus, several of these pressures are a direct byproduct of behavior you can do something about.

The items below came directly from senior executives in national and regional health insurance companies. They asked for anonymity, as they are either still working in these organizations or don't want to face market blowback.

Pressure to Include Less Desirable Hospitals in Networks

This is caused by pressure from employers to have every possible provider in their network so their employees don't complain about lack of choice. Of course, having every provider means that you have lower and higher-quality providers in the same network. This also means higher costs because the lower-quality providers are generally less efficient and deliver improper, excessive, or low-value care, which leads to complications, overtreatment, and even death. Data showing this is generally very reliable, despite claims from those scoring poorly; every day, it gets more so.

In addition, contracts between insurance carriers and hospitals in some regions include anti-steerage language. This language requires the insurer to include a given health system network in all of its plans. For example, in northern California, UnitedHealth might have an agreement with Sutter Health that prevents them from excluding Sutter from any employer agreement. The Affordable Care Act (ACA) made this worse by allowing hospitals to aggregate in ways that enable oligopolistic practices.

Plus, employers often seek to include their local hospital and every physician in-network to minimize employee complaints, regardless of the hospital's or physician's quality (or cost).

Poor Service from Carriers Is a Natural Byproduct of Medical Loss Ratio Rules

This is a direct effect of the ACA. Because of the Medical Loss Ratio prescribed in the ACA, it requires that 80 or 85 percent of premiums be spent on medical care (depending on type of plan), and carriers are forced to cut customer service employees for fully-insured plans—considered overhead—to escape penalties under the ACA. This is exacerbated as companies move from fully-insured to self-insured status (in part to escape ACA regulations). Because customer service functions are often shared across fully-insured and self-insured business, the lower-margin self-insured business puts further pressure on carriers to find cost savings. Generally, self-insured plans have less than 10 percent the profit opportunity of fully-insured plans.[66]

In addition, Medical Loss Ratio requirements cap insurance company profits, meaning that the only practical ways to increase profits is to reduce service staff, raise premiums, or process more claims.

New Fees to Replace Lost Margin

The co-dependent relationship between insurance carriers and hospitals is evident with out-of-network charges. Remember, when health systems impose egregious out-of-network charges, insurers are happy to pay them immediately and with no review whatsoever (and with your money), because it generates more revenue for them in a number of ways. Naturally, they can't say this. Plus, employers have been haranguing them for decades any time an employee complains about any delayed or denied claim or balance bill from a care provider. So, in response to this profit incentive and to give you what your benefits managers ask for, they sell this as a benefit for you: You and your employees won't be bothered by hospital collections departments!

They follow paying the ridiculous out-of-network charges with "re-pricing" that discounts charges to seemingly more reasonable levels—on your behalf, of course. What may not be clear is that the insurance carrier gets paid 30-40 percent of the repriced claim. This encourages the hospital to push the pre-discount prices ever higher, which pushes the discount up and, with it, the fee paid by the employer and net amount of each claim. Of course, we all pay in the end via increased costs and premiums.

Another fee opportunity is so-called "pay and chase" programs, in which the insurance carrier doing your claims administration gets paid 30-40 percent for recovering fraudulent or duplicative claims. Thus, there is a perverse incentive to tacitly allow fraudulent and duplicative claims to be paid, get paid as the plan administrator, then get paid a second time for recovering the originally paid claim.

Many of the fraud prevention tools used by claims administrators are laughably outdated and weak compared to what they are up against. Modern payment integrity solutions can stop fraud and duplicate claims, but aren't being used by most self-insured companies' claims administrators. In a report on fraud, Accenture found that "estimates by government and law enforcement agencies, such as the FBI, place the loss due to health care fraud as high as 10 percent of annual health care expenditure."[67] This is roughly $300 billion per year! Payment integrity experts, such as Dave Adams, CEO of 4C Health Solutions, tell me stories of companies that have paid the same claim 25-50 times because the claims administrator didn't use modern tools to stop it.

Many times, they don't do anything about it. Other times they do a bill review and try to recover those monies, getting the "pay and chase" recovery payment.

It's worth noting again that employee behavior is often a primary root cause of these practices. Whenever employees get a bill from a care provider as a result of a denied claim, they complain to your HR department or broker, who, in turn, complains to the insurance carrier, leading them to give your company what you ask for. As with most dysfunction in health care, simple incentives and behaviors often have enormous, counterintuitive, and costly consequences.

Dancing the Frustrating Kabuki Dance

Why does an insurance carrier give you a renewal rate and then keep reducing it until you bite, especially when you're fully-insured? Because the insurance carrier makes ten times more on premiums from fully-insured clients than on fees from self-insured clients.[68] As a result, insurance executives face enormous pressure to keep and grow their fully-insured books of business. Bonuses and other incentives for benefits brokers and consultants to keep business with the same carrier cement this dynamic. Increasingly, carriers even offer early renewals to keep fully-insured business. Often these early renewals come with no-shop clauses. So, a 20 percent rate increase may only be 15 percent if you sign today and agree not to shop the competition. This should be viewed as a red-flag, not a great deal on a premium reduction. The first thing to do if you ever get a no-shop offer is to warm up the RFPs and start shopping.

Your Claims Data Somehow Belongs to the Insurance Carrier

Amazingly, insurance carriers have convinced employers to accept that their own claims data are proprietary to the carrier—and they refuse to share them. Equally amazingly, employers often agree to contract terms that severely limit their access to audit claims, often being able to audit just a tiny subset.

There are only three reasons insurance carriers would claim the data is proprietary.

1. Their reporting and data systems are so poor that they literally can't share. This is much less likely these days.
2. If they release the data, a good actuary consultant could dive in and raise lots of questions they don't want to answer. For example, they could see that an organization pays a large multiple of market pricing or has questionably high use of a particular test or procedure.
3. They want to maintain the status quo. This means protecting pricing opacity at all costs. If you could see the prices you actually pay, you might begin to wonder why a hospital with a large market share but mediocre quality outcomes is paid exponentially more than a smaller, high-quality provider in the same network.

It should be clear that numbers two and three are more likely. Hospitals and insurance carriers want to avoid defending or explaining pricing and the various fees they bake in. This largely comes from the pressure insurance and hospital executives face to keep growing profits by 10 to 15 percent year over year.

Inflated Health Care Cost Trends

Insurance executives are under huge pressure to grow their business, even with self-insured accounts. One way insurance carriers try to prevent independent third-party plan administrators from winning employer business is inflating the medical trend (the rate at which health care costs are increasing) for their fully-insured clients by one percent. This additional money is then used to create bonuses (override programs) for benefits brokers, workplace wellness programs, and broker implementation credits (additional payments for help rolling out a program) as incentives for winning or maintaining fully-insured and self-insured clients. Think of this as robbing Peter, unknowingly, to pay Paul. As a result, fully-insured clients are cross-subsidizing low-value workplace wellness programs or paying to fund broker override programs that do not impact them at all.

Broker Incentives that Preserve Status Quo Inertia

Insurance carriers often have programs that require a broker to maintain a 90 percent retention rate to receive a year-end bonus. These programs help carriers retain clients and can be $300,000 to $500,000 for each local office of a brokerage. This amount often represents most of the net profit for an office and can heavily influence brokers who might otherwise advise you to move to a self-insured plan. Because bonuses are based on the total business a particular broker brings to an insurance carrier, they typically aren't included in the list of claims costs, commissions, or fees, unless the broker has a transparent practice—which most don't. If it seems like your broker makes your current carrier's renewal plan look better than other options, this is probably why. You should ask if he or she gets paid any bonuses from particular carriers. To simplify this, Appendix C has a disclosure form you can use to understand your broker's overall financial incentives and potential conflicts before making a purchasing decision.[69]

In short, the broker you treat as your buyer's agent is actually compensated as a seller's agent, creating a conflict you wouldn't accept in other contexts.

Carriers and Brokers Are Soft on Area Hospitals

When your insurance carrier also administers the health plan for hospital employees or your broker represents the hospital, there are additional forces working against you. Hospitals are often one of the larger employers in a town or region, so the insurance carrier won't risk losing them as a client. Since the hospital provides a large revenue stream, the carrier typically goes easy on them when negotiating pricing on behalf of other clients—like you. Additionally, some brokers get as much as 30 percent of their revenue from hospitals and other care providers.

You should always ask your benefits broker or claims administrator if a local hospital is a client, as that is a clear conflict of interest, especially when the hospital itself owns the insurance carrier.

State Mandates

One benefit of self-insuring is avoiding state mandates and regulatory requirements that apply to fully-insured plans and that can meaningfully increase your overall costs. This benefit disappears if your insurance carrier incorporates these mandates into their self-insured plan offerings, even when they weren't intended for an organization like yours. Why would they do that? Different treatment of different business lines and employer accounts creates complexity that insurance carriers want to avoid. Logical and efficient for them, costly for you.

Key Take-aways

- Despite perceptions, insurance companies usually go easy on hospitals, especially if they do a lot of business with them.
- Beware if one of your service providers, such as a benefits broker or insurance company, has a hospital as one of their biggest customers.
- The data your service provider won't let you see belongs to you, and the lack of visibility is hurting you.
- New fees constantly get snuck in. Question everything.

CHAPTER 6

HEALTH CARE IS STEALING MILLENNIALS' FUTURE - BUT THEY WILL TAKE IT BACK

"We can't solve problems by using the same kind of thinking we used when we created them." – Albert Einstein

If we can't slay the health care beast, millennials will see their future stolen from them. As the largest generation in history and now the largest chunk of the workforce (see Figure 6), they will make their presence felt.

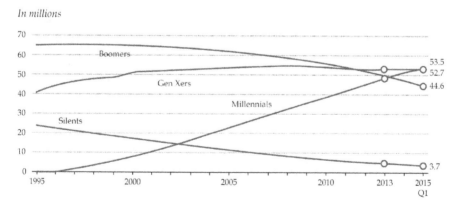

Figure 6. Source: Richard Fry, "Millennials Surpass Gen Xers as the Largest Generation in U.S. Labor Force," Pew Research Center, (July 4th, 2016).[70]

Whether through government favoring the largest special interest groups (e.g., hospitals, pharmaceutical companies, and insurance companies) rather than the people or through self-inflicted mistakes (e.g., the HMO "gatekeeper" and denial of care debacle), health care has been remarkably resilient to forces trying to disrupt it for decades—forces that have driven change in virtually every other sector from financial services to retail to travel. Millennials will bring this disruption to health care.

Becky and Her Biggest Expense

If you only read one (other) book about health care, read David Goldhill's *Catastrophic Care: Why Everything We Think We Know about Health Care Is Wrong*. Formerly CFO of a large media organization, Goldhill is currently CEO of The Game Show Network. He also lost his father to a hospital-acquired infection and saw numerous errors during that hospitalization. This experience caused him to bring his financial acumen to health care. If he didn't break it down with well-sourced figures, Goldhill's conclusions would be unbelievable. Who could imagine that during their adult lives, one out of every two dollars earned by millennials will go to a health care system that is the perfect polar opposite to what they want and value? That is, if the current trajectory isn't altered. Keep in mind that, while well over 80 percent of health-related spending goes to the "sick care" system, that system only drives 20 percent of health outcomes.

Figure 7 tells a terrifying story, but more shocking is how conservative the assumptions behind the numbers are. The following description of these assumptions is from Goldhill's book.

Share of Lifetime Earnings of a Millennial That Will Go to Health Care Unless We Change Course

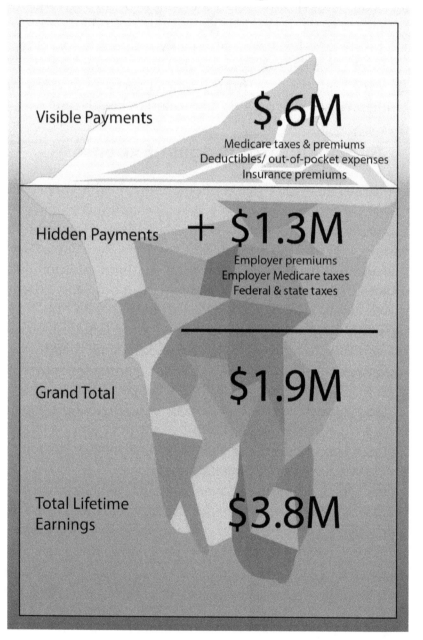

Figure 7. Source: Numbers come from Goldhill's book and are over the course of a millennial's lifetime.[71]

Let's give this millennial a name, Becky, and make a few assumptions about her life. We'll say she gets married at 30 and has two children. She works until she's 65 and dies at 80. We'll also assume her income grows every year by 4 percent, so that at retirement she's earning $180,000 a year. To simplify the analysis, we'll have Becky's husband leave her to join an ashram when he turns 65, so she's only responsible for her own Medicare premiums. Let's also give Becky a stroke of good fortune and say that she and her dependents stay healthy, with no major health crisis requiring large out-of-pocket expenditures.

Now allow me to make a truly crazy assumption just for the sake of argument. Let's assume that health care costs grow at only two percent a year—half of Becky's income growth. This hasn't been true for forty-five years, but we can always hope. Given all those factors, how much do you think Becky will contribute to the health care system for herself and her dependents over her lifetime? I'll give you a hint: Becky will earn $3.85 million over her career. The answer is $1.9 million! If she has a working spouse, the two will contribute $2.5 million into this system over their lifetimes.[72]

How has this happened? Remember that Becky is almost certainly unaware of how many ways she is paying into the health care system, even though she'll probably put more into that system than she spends on anything else over her entire life.

This projection takes on added urgency when you consider that obesity rates have tripled among young adults in the past three decades, from eight percent in 1971-1974 to 24 percent in 2005- 2006, thanks to the diet of what Michael Pollan calls "food-like substances" that their Boomer parents fed them. This is causing millennials to engage more broadly in the health care system much earlier than previous generations. As Figure 8 shows, only 20 percent of health outcomes are the result of clinical care. The areas that represent the other 80 percent are a good place to start for understanding where millennials will likely take our health care system. Finally, the jig is up. A do-it-yourself health reform movement is rising—and not a moment too soon. Solutions are coming from the edges: from forward-looking employers, innovative towns, fed up physicians, and, especially, from millennials wising up. Ask any venture capitalist whom they study to get insight into the future and they'll give you a clear answer—millennials.

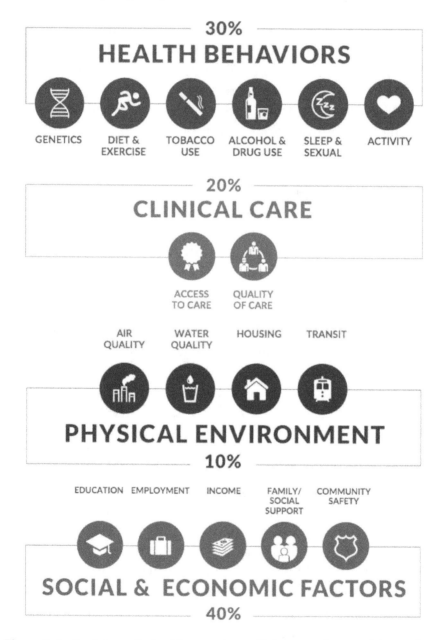

Figure 8. In the future, the health ecosystem will focus on the true drivers of outcomes, of which clinical care is only 20 percent.[73]

Millennials to the Rescue

Millennials, people 20-36 in 2018, have driven society-wide change in many areas. Their early adoption of technology made smartphones, social media, and services such as Uber pervasive across all generations. That row of empty storefronts in your town? That's the power of millennials.

Financial services is a good example of millennials steering the market away from today's market leaders.[74] Well-known brand strategist Adam Hanft, author of *The Stunning Evolution of Millennials: They've Become the Ben Franklin Generation*, could have been talking about health care when he wrote:

> *[Millennials'] faith in technology is understandable. Algorithms don't act in their own self-interest. Algorithms weren't responsible for dreaming up sub-prime loans and nearly bringing down the financial system. Millennials didn't trust authority and conventional sources of wisdom before the melt-down. Imagine now. Wealthfront argues that millennials: '…have been nickel-and-dimed through a wide variety of services, and they value simple, transparent, low-cost services.'[75]*

> *Millennials have also driven the growth of Wealthfront, an alternative to traditional financial advisers who frequently steer clients toward their own firm's financial products. In contrast, Wealthfront has mimicked, in algorithmic form, the portfolio investment strategies of the most sophisticated wealth managers (e.g., rebalancing portfolios, tax-loss harvesting), traditionally available only to very high net worth individuals.*

Hanft goes on to offer a word of warning to the financial industry that could just as easily be applied to the health care industry. "The giants of financial service haven't seen the [volcanic] shifts that travel, media, entertainment and home thermostats have. They will. Depending on who you are, the Ben Franklin generation is composed of 80 million Benedict Arnolds."

Industry giants may want to ignore this trend, but millennials are the canary in the coal mine, because the fact is everyone wants these features. As Danny Chrichton, a venture capitalist investor at CRV—and a millennial—has said, "consumers want to be able to manage their finances from their phones and tablets while limiting their visits to bank branches and bank tellers. Plus, everyone hates bank fees, particularly their complexity and lack of transparency. The difference is that millennials are willing to shop elsewhere, because we are simply not going to accept that these are the only products on the market."[76]

Another example of millennials forcing change is the newspaper industry. Millennials ignored newspapers as a source of news but also as the de facto place to buy/sell items. (Craigslist anyone?). Undermining classified ads, which were roughly half of newspaper profits, made newspapers a demonstrably worse product. Those profits previously supported the reporting that has declined sharply over the last 10 years. Many papers have even had to eliminate editions on some days, further accelerating the trend.

Health Care Priorities: Cost and Convenience

The health system parallels to newspaper classified ads are profit centers such as cardiac catheterization labs—sometimes nicknamed "cash labs," as they are also centers of overuse. Cardiac catheterization led to the development of wonderful interventions—angioplasty, coronary artery bypass grafts, stents—that revolutionized cardiology in the 20th century. Without question, this saved lives. But the fact that these procedures are grossly overused is no longer in question either.

Overuse in health care is not simply a matter of wasted resources, money, and time. It exposes patients to terrible harm—often including death. Here's what happened to one 52-year-old woman who came into an ER with chest pain after starting a new exercise regime. Shannon Brownlee, Senior Vice President of the Lown Institute, described the situation at the Health Care

Town Hall Meeting at the Frontier Cafe in Brunswick, Maine on November 6, 2014:

"The emergency doctor thought it was almost certainly a pulled muscle, but just to be sure he ordered a new and special CT scan of the heart. It showed a little something, as these scans so often do, and so just to be sure he sent her to the cath lab. There was nothing wrong with her heart until they perforated her aorta. They did an emergency bypass from which she recovered; but then she had graft bypass rejection and she had to have her heart replaced. This is a person who came into the emergency room with a pulled muscle."

Cath labs are no longer the sound investment they once were. Millennials, more than previous generations, want to know all the diagnostic and treatment possibilities when they're sick or injured and are more likely to select lower-cost, less invasive treatment options. This is also what most people of all generations want when given full information. Again, millennials are just the drivers.

Given their insistence on new ways of doing business on every front, it's not surprising that millennials are avoiding the ill-designed norms in health care. For example, selecting a doctor. It's not that millennials aren't loyal to their physicians when convenient, but they're far more willing than boomers to "doctor shop" until they are satisfied. They're looking for same-day appointments, online scheduling, easy access to their medical records, and the option to text or email the doctor between visits, according to KQED's Chrissy Farr.[77]

The vast majority of people who use ZocDoc—a website that helps individuals schedule doctor's visits—are millennials. Many of the doctors who have signed up on ZocDoc offer text and email communication, as well as weekend and evening appointments.

Retail clinics, typically found in national pharmacy chains like Walgreens and CVS, are another innovation being embraced by cost- and convenience-conscious millennials. Between 2006 and 2014, the number of retail clinics in the United States grew from 200 to 1,800, while visits grew sevenfold to 1.5 million.[78]

A PNC health care survey found that 34 percent of people ages 18 to 34 prefer retail clinics—about double the rate of 17 percent for baby boomers and 15 percent for older seniors.[79]

New Benefits Choices for Smart Communities

Millennials may be more interested than their parents in getting the most for their health care dollar, but nearly three in four of them are confused about their benefit options, according to a 2016 Harris Poll. And almost half would rather clean out their email than research those options.[80]

Why is this important to you and your company? Because that same survey shows that 76 percent of millennials say health care benefits strongly factor in their decision about where to work.[81]

Millennials are now the biggest portion of the workforce and will be 75 percent of it in 12 years.[82] The time has come for benefits brokers to fulfill their promise and guide their clients toward developing new benefits programs optimized for millennials.

For example, smart employers can shift their workforce to a higher-performing benefits package through tiers that introduce changes. Under this strategy, the old "get less, pay more" status quo package becomes "Tier 2." The new benefits offering is "Tier 1" and is the default package for new employees.

Freelancers now make up 35% of U.S. workers and collectively earned $1 trillion in 2016.[83] That translates to 55 million people. While these aren't all millennials, the newly named CEO of the Amazon – Berkshire Hathaway – JP Morgan Chase health organization spoke to the imperative to fill this need. During an interview with PBS' Judy Woodruff,[84] Dr. Atul Gawande stated, "Tying how you get your health care to your place of employment is going to become less and less tenable as fewer and fewer people are getting coverage through employment. We miss this important statistic. Larry Katz and a team show this. Over the last

10 years (data was from 2005-2015) 94% of net new job growth was in forms of employment that had no health care benefits. It was alternative work forms. It was gig employment, independent contracting, temporary workers. That's the world my kids are now walking into. When they get their employment, they are most likely to be in that category."

As outlined in Chapter 19, forward-looking mayors are embracing Economic Development 3.0 mindset. Increasingly millennials are choosing where they want to work geographically, before they choose the specific company or job they'll choose. Mayors, such as Lauren Poe of Gainesville, Florida, are actively working to make their communities more attractive by ensuring there are great health benefits options that go beyond typical ACA plans that mean many people are functionally uninsured when the majority of U.S. households have less than $1,000 in savings. That is, if you have a bronze or silver plan, the average deductible is $5,873 and $3,937 respectively.[85] In other words, even while technically being insured, you are a bad stubbed toe away from financial ruin.

This is the millennials' moment. They're not alone, but will suffer the devastating consequences of an out-of-control health care system more than anyone. When millennials rise to the occasion, I believe they'll be remembered as the Greatest Generation of the 21st century.

Key Take-aways

- On the current path, millennials would become indentured servants to the health care system, spending half to two-thirds of lifetime earnings on health care. Millennials will ensure that never happens, which will drive tremendous change in health benefits unlike we have ever seen.
- We all ultimately desire what millennials desire, whether it's smart phones, better food, social media, or better health care.
- As health care change will happen in phases, millennials are natural early adopters of greatly improved health care.

ROSEN HOTELS & RESORTS

Smart Benefits Lead to Huge Gains in Education Outcomes and Crime Reduction

In my experience, speaking with many employers who have slayed the health care cost beast, there has been one recurring theme: A leader took the bull by the horns—and did so knowing that success involves weaving employees into the reinvention process rather than trying to pull the wool over their eyes.

Harris Rosen is the founder, COO, and president of Rosen Hotels & Resorts, a small regional chain in Orlando, Florida. Though he's not a health care expert, he intuitively knew what PwC data famously showed: half of health care spending doesn't add value.[86] In a business of ups and downs in which staff costs are a major factor, Rosen surrounded himself with a special executive team to tackle this challenge.

To date, they've adopted more Health Rosetta components than any other company I know, saving approximately $315 million on health care costs since 1971 and spending 50 percent less per capita than the average employer. If all employers followed suit, we could conservatively remove $500 billion of waste from health care and shift it to more productive sectors of the economy.

Their plan has also grown from 500 to 5,700 lives as the company has grown. They have a very culturally, racially, socioeconomically, and demographically diverse employee base, including many immigrants who often haven't had regular access to care before. Yet single coverage for the average employee is only $18.75 per week for benefits that include medical, dental, and pharmacy and, as you'll see below, are better than most of us have ever had.

Rosen also uses focus groups and surveys to match up programs with employee needs, and they continuously refine their programs. Here are a few elements of what makes their program successful:

- They have a comprehensive, onsite, 12,000-sf medical center that provides access to many routine health care services, far more than typical primary care. They furnished it with used but modern and functional medical equipment for 10 to 15 cents on the dollar. Employees are able to visit the center "on the clock," thus removing a major barrier to receiving care.
- They take great care of individuals, hiring health coaches and nurses to serve as coaches and navigators throughout a medical journey. They use robust, evidence-based approaches to case management, inpatient care management, care transitions, and medication compliance management.
- They have eschewed the blunt instrument approaches most employers use to cut costs (high copays, deductibles) in favor of $5 office visit copays, zero copays for 90 percent of pharmaceuticals, and no co-insurance. Where necessary, they offer free transportation to appointments to further remove barriers to care.
- Company events serve food approved by nutritionists and the director of health services. They also offer cooking courses.
- They offer the most effective kind of wellness programs for free, including onsite stretching and exercise (e.g., Zumba, kick-boxing, walking programs, spinning, boot camp), flu shots and vaccinations, family planning, educational materials, nutritional services, and health fairs and physicals on a

schedule informed by the U.S. Preventive Services Task Force, which is far more conservative than the one workplace wellness vendors push.

- They provide free health screenings for colon cancer, diabetes, breast cancer (onsite mammograms), high cholesterol, hypertension, and sexually transmitted diseases, along with visits from registered dietitians. Furthermore, this program is based on evidence-based guidelines from organizations like the U.S. Preventive Services Task Force to minimize misdiagnosis and overtreatment.
- Despite physically demanding jobs, onsite physical therapy has led to opioid prescription rates that are one-sixth of the national average.
- They have a mandatory stretching program for housekeepers and other employees with a higher risk of injury, reducing injuries by 25 percent.
- Fifty-six percent of their employees' pregnancies are high risk as a result of high rates of advanced maternal age, diabetes, hypertension, and HIV. The company is very proactive about helping employees manage pregnancies (a premature birth can cost $500,000).
- The company cafeteria provides discounts for healthier foods to reduce consumption of unhealthier foods, e.g., discounts on salads. The dietitian and director of health services analyze employee cafeteria offerings for portion size and nutritional benefit. They also use signage to educate employees about nutrition, use smaller plates to control portion sizes, and limit fried food.
- They focus on better management of chronic conditions and have even seen a drop in development of new chronic conditions. This is especially important for workers coming from developing countries who often have complex diseases.

Rosen is partnering with other businesses in their community to expand this approach, demonstrating that it's worth ruffling a few feathers to gain the dual benefit of lower costs and a healthier, more satisfied workforce. The ripple effects extend well beyond the company, boosting employee well-being and their broader community's economy. For example, in an industry that sees employee turnover approaching 60 percent, Rosen has turnover in the low teens.

Rosen pays for full-time employees' college tuition after 5 years of employment. They also pay state college tuition for employees' children after just 3 years of employment.

They've also used money that would have been overspent on health care to fuel a range of creative philanthropy. Rosen started by paying for preschool in the underserved, once crime-ridden Tangelo Park neighborhood in Orlando. He's also continued to fund various programs to help those kids develop, such as paying for their college education in full (tuition, room/board, and books). The results have been breathtaking.

- Crime has been reduced by 63 percent.
- High school graduation rates went from 45 percent to nearly 100 percent.
- College graduation rates are 77 percent above the national average.

The cost over 24 years of the Tangelo Park program has been $11 million—roughly the amount Rosen saves in one year on health care. Recently Rosen has agreed to adopt another underserved community called Parramore, which is five times the size of Tangelo Park.

For Harris Rosen, the approach is simple: Get involved; care for your people.

Key Take-aways

- Managing health care costs, like any other big expense, reaps huge dividends.
- For every high cost area, there's a sound approach that overachieves on Quadruple Aim objectives.
- Money no longer squandered on health care can change a community – whether that community is a community of employees or a neighborhood.

Part II

How and Why We Are Getting Fleeced

The health care industry has been extremely deft at persuading us to accept hyperinflating costs we wouldn't accept in any other area of our lives. In this part of the book, we highlight the most common ways the industry ensures that their revenue and profits grow inexorably and we delve into three of the biggest areas that are least understood.

For example, it would be logical to assume that an insurance company could aggregate their buying power to get your organization a better deal. While this certainly is possible and can happen to an extent, just the opposite generally happens. The much-vaunted PPO networks actually ensure that you pay for the privilege of greatly overpaying for health care services. Then there's criminal fraud. While it's impossible not to know about cybercrime and cybersecurity issues, most leaders don't know that as much as 10 percent of all claims their organization pays are fraudulent due to a lack of oversight. Finally, we debunk the notion that workplace wellness programs will have any demonstrable impact on costs. While there may be reasons to have workplace wellness programs, cost reduction isn't one of them.

7 TRICKS USED TO REDISTRIBUTE MONEY FROM YOUR ORGANIZATION TO THE HEALTH CARE INDUSTRY

"There are two primary choices in life: to accept conditions as they exist, or accept the responsibility for changing them."– Denis Waitley

The health care industry has been remarkably effective at extracting as much money as possible from the U.S. economy. Employers and individuals pick up the majority of this tab.[87] Unlike virtually every other item in our economy, where the value proposition improves every year, the norm in health care for decades has been to pay more and get less. Also, unlike nearly every other industry, health care hasn't had a productivity gain in 20 years.[88]

In other words, for the last two decades, there has been a redistribution "tax" from the working and middle class and highly efficient industries to the least productive industry in America.[89] Here's what you need to know to emulate savvy leaders who have already addressed the issues described below.

Costly Health Care Industry Tricks

This list is not exhaustive but does highlight some of the largest cost issues. Once you know what to look for, you can reverse course by applying the strategies and lessons from Parts III and IV of this book.

While these tricks exist in both fully-insured and self-insured organizations, the ability to take corrective action is largely limited to self-insured organizations. Understanding that fully-insured employers already bear much of the risk of being self-insured, but without the benefits, helps simplify the decision to go self-insured. If you're a fully-insured employer and have higher-than-expected claims in one year, your insurance carrier will work to get as much back as possible in subsequent years through larger premium increases.

Employers with well-managed plans are already reducing health benefits spending by 20 percent or more with better results—directing savings toward higher and better uses.

And let me say before we plunge into the dark side of health care that there are many, many exceptional health care organizations and professionals—insurance carriers, plan administrators, benefits brokers, physicians, hospitals, nursing homes—that don't employ these unethical practices. Plus, a vanguard of doctors and others are leading the way to stamp out the bad actors for good.

Trick #1: Directing Patients to the Most Expensive Treatment Options, Even If They're Not the Most Effective

People often raise the specter of rationing care. In reality, it's overuse (i.e., unnecessary and potentially harmful care) that leads to reduced access by squandering enormous financial resources that would be better used for individuals who actually need care and can't get it.

I asked Garrison Bliss, MD, the founder of the first direct primary care practice—a model for employers and individuals to directly contract with primary care clinicians in high-value, cost-reducing arrangements—how they were able to achieve a 30 to 50 percent reduction in surgeries. The answer was remarkably simple: Let people choose.

For example, one of the most common reasons people go to the doctor is back pain, one of the most overtreated symptoms around. Having personally experienced searing back pain, I would do almost anything to make it go away. If I'm told that surgery and opioids are the only way to go, that's what I'll probably do. However, it turns out that physical therapy is very often more effective than surgery. According to Bliss, individuals will virtually always choose the least invasive and safest treatments when they're clearly told about the pros and cons of potential options.

This doesn't typically happen though. A primary reason is that hospital-employed primary care doctors receive financial incentives to refer patients to high-margin specialty practices. In Chapter 11, we'll learn that 90 percent of back surgeries performed at Virginia Mason Hospital & Medical Center were unnecessary and that musculoskeletal (MSK) procedures account for roughly 20 percent of all health care spending. By simply deploying an evidence-based MSK program, a large tire manufacturer improved its earnings by 1.7 percent; had it been able to get all of its employees who have MSK issues into the program, its positive earnings impact could have been five percent. How many corporate initiatives can increase earnings by five percent?

Trick #2: Turning Primary Care into a Milk-in-the-Back-of-the-Store Loss Leader

Dr. Paul Grundy, IBM's chief medical officer and director of health care transformation, shared with me how his company undertook a two-year study from 2005-2006 of its $2 billion annual global health care spent. The results reinforced what many already knew—there is a strong bias against primary care that has been highly effective at undermining this valuable resource in favor of higher-cost specialty care. One consequence of this is the 10-minute primary care appointment, which leaves little time to delve into the root cause of whatever issues bring an individual to the office. This pressures physicians to take short-cuts to satisfying patients—ordering a test or prescribing a drug. This pattern is also a key driver of the opioid crisis, as are well-intended patient satisfaction surveys that feature questions about the patient's happiness with the pain control measures they were given. A provider's scores on these surveys is an increasingly significant factor in how much they're reimbursed for government-sponsored programs like Medicare.

Trick #3: Using Intentionally Bewildering and Absurd Drug Pricing

Drug pricing, which accounts for an increasingly large share of your benefits spending, is bewildering by design. It's part of the strategy to get away with exorbitant prices. Pharmacy Benefit Management (PBM) firms are well-known for hidden fees, shell game pricing, and taking drug manufacturers' money to promote specific medications.[90] With the breathtaking spike in specialty drug prices in recent years, these practices are costing all of us dearly.

Recently, two very well-known PBMs added a brand drug called Duexis to their formularies, which currently sells for more than $4,000 for a 90-day supply. Duexis is a combination of two drugs you may have in your medicine cabinet that together cost only a few bucks—ibuprofen and famotidine (common household names, Motrin and Pepcid). Vimovo is another expensive combination drug that is just delayed-release omeprazole (Prilosec) and naproxen sodium (Aleve).

PBM consultant CrystalClearRx pulled data to show the drastic difference in pricing for a 90-day supply of these two brand drugs and their generic counterparts at the same dosage.[91]

Duexis	Ibuprofen+Famotidine
$4,680	$20 to $40
Vimovo	**Omeprazole + Naproxen Sodium**
$2,279	$20 to $40

In these cases, the brand drugs are 50 to 234 times more expensive for functionally the same drug. PBMs are incentivized to add these kinds of drugs to formularies so they can tout big discounts off high-cost drug costs. It also lets them capture high-margin revenue from hidden rebates they receive from drug manufacturers. Rebates are a form of arbitrage where PBMs receive money back on each claim for a particular drug. They typically either don't refund this to you at all or only partially refund it.

PBMs are also sometimes owned by insurance carriers but are not held to the margin requirements the ACA imposes on the carrier. The PBM reaps enormous profits, while allowing the carrier to cry "poor" and raise your rates.

Enough said.

Trick #4: Not Suggesting Management Strategies for Rare but Astronomical Claims

Benefits manager Tom Emerick, co-author of *Cracking Health Costs: How to Cut Your Company's Health Costs and Provide Employees Better Care*, pointed out how outlier claims are the biggest driver of the health care cost explosion. During his career, Emerick typically found that six percent of employees in a given year accounted for 80 percent of company medical costs. So, he set up a Centers of Excellence program to address the most expensive cases: employees and family members needing heart, spine, and transplant surgeries are sent to six of the most highly rated and thus most cost-effective health care organizations in the country for free care—if they need it.

Often, they don't. Emerick's book explains how his largest

employer found that 40 percent of planned organ transplants at local hospitals were deemed medically unnecessary when their employees visited top notch providers such as Mayo Clinic for a second opinion. In a study published in 2017, Mayo Clinic reported that as many as 88 percent of patients who visit the clinic for a second opinion on a complex procedure go home with a new or refined diagnosis—changing their care plan and potentially saving their lives.

Dialysis management is another source of extraordinary bills. More than 25,000,000 Americans have chronic kidney disease, and 100,000 start dialysis each year. This is inevitable, but employers can turn the huge disparity among costs for the same service, from $100,000 to more than $500,000, to their advantage by scouting out the lowest-cost, high-quality services.

Trick #5: Hiding the Use of Accessory—and Often Out-of-Network—Physicians

It happens all the time: You have the insurance carrier's authorization for your physician, who is part of your plan's PPO network, to perform a procedure like a surgery or colonoscopy. Everything seems straightforward—until you get the bill and see charges from an anesthetist, a pathologist, or a radiologist you don't know and who turns out to be out-of-network; this means he or she is not subject to negotiated discounts and will require larger out-of-pocket fees from you.

This is what happened to Gap Inc. and it had much larger consequences than just paying more for care. Their HR leaders have been named in a lawsuit for breach of fiduciary duty for not applying proper care in managing their health plan.[92] (See Chapter 26 for more discussion of employer fiduciary responsibilities issues under ERISA.) Some employers have tried to head off this situation with much touted "wrap networks," designed primarily to cover employees who need care when they're away from home. But the wrap network rates are typically significantly higher than the rates under your PPO network. And it may actually cost more to file a claim under a wrap network than to have your benefits administrator negotiate a disputed claim (a service offered by modern TPAs).

Trick #6: Delivering Inappropriate Oncology Treatment

Sadly, way too much cancer treatment is unproven. Cancer centers may not follow evidence-based treatment guidelines for certain cancers and too often have limited regard for the devastating side effects patients experience during and after treatment. Also, financial conflicts are rampant at cancer centers, which may not inform individuals and their families about costs, copayments, and co-insurance before treatment.

Dr. Otis Brawley, MD, chief medical officer for the American Cancer Society and author of *How We Do Harm: A Doctor Breaks Ranks about Being Sick in America,* famously said that "the talk should not be about rationing care but about rational health care." He described taking over the care of a patient with colon cancer who was dumped by his doctor after losing his insurance. Dr. Brawley found that the patient was on a chemotherapy regimen that was 15 years out of date and taking unnecessary drugs on which the first doctor was receiving a substantial markup.

"I've seen so many times," wrote Brawley, "where doctors really have failed to evolve and… learn as the profession and the scientific evidence have changed over time."[93]

Putting his experience in context, the *BMJ Quality and Safety Journal* has estimated that 28 percent of cancers are misdiagnosed in the first place.[94]

Trick #7: Suppressing Quality and Safety Data

Not only is it statistically safer to be in an airplane than a hospital, it's also statistically 47x safer to deliberately jump *out* of that plane as a skydiver than to be in a hospital.[95] Surprised? That's just how the health care industry wants it.

Industry lobbying power—and health care lobbyists outspend the oil, financial, and defense industries *combined*—is on full display when it comes to hiding quality and safety information from the public.[96] Fortunately, other people are determined to dig that information out and get it to you.

Leapfrog, an independent nonprofit founded by leading employers and health care experts, promotes health care transparency through data collection and public reporting initiatives. You can check Leapfrog Hospital Safety Grades online for your local hospitals.[97] Their quality grades are based on a voluntary annual hospital survey they conduct, but only around 1,800 of 5,564 U.S. hospitals currently participate. Leapfrog also publishes safety grades based on publicly available data and the survey results for participating hospitals.

You can also go to Medicare's Hospital Compare, which provides data on the 4,000+ hospitals that are Medicare-certified, to find out how hospitals in your area are performing on some 60 measures, everything from serious complication rates to the percent of patients who report being given information about what to do after discharge and during recovery.[98]

In addition, you can find safety and other data about physicians at Vitals.com, RateMDs.com, and HealthGrades.com.

None of these ratings efforts are entirely satisfactory, some less so than others, but it's a start. More important, you can ask questions. As an employer, it's your job to find out as much as you can about the care available to your employees and you have the ability to do so—no matter what the industry says.

Key Take-aways

- The dominant primary care model prevalent in the U.S. is designed to get you as quickly as possible to costly procedures and tests that favor the health care system revenue rather than health outcomes.

- PBMs design formularies to push brand drugs that cost 100 times more than equally-effective generics and over-the-counter drugs, so they can optimize their bottom line.
- Complex medical situations are often misdiagnosed and addressed by health systems with inadequate experience and/or improper safety procedures, with severe health and financial consequences.

CHAPTER 8

PPO NETWORKS DELIVER VALUE—AND OTHER FLAWED ASSUMPTIONS THAT CRUSH YOUR BUDGET

"Your assumptions are your windows on the world. Scrub them off every once in a while, or the light won't come in." – Isaac Asimov

Albert Einstein famously said, "We can't solve problems by using the same kind of thinking we used when we created them." Yet, this is exactly what health care does over and over. Baked into our thinking about health benefits administration are many assumptions that turn out to be flawed on deeper examination—at best outdated, at worst outrageous.

Here are three flawed assumptions that are doing you serious harm.

1. Your broker works for you*

There are certainly some excellent brokers that do their best for employers, but the overwhelming majority have undisclosed conflicts of interest that favor insurance carriers. In this book, the term benefits consultant or advisor refers to people who provide a broader range of services and expertise than simply signing up clients on behalf of a carrier. Many of them bring a more sophisticated brand of professionalism to their clients. See Chapter 13 – 7 habits for a more complete treatment of this critical subject.

2. Insurance carriers want to drive down costs and PPO networks deliver the best pricing available
3. Auto-adjudication of claims is always good

Together, these assumptions may seem minor, but together they add up to significant costs and damage to your bottom line, your employees' bottom line, and your employees' health. Luckily, knowing about them is half the battle to counter acting them.

Flawed Assumption #1: Your Broker Works for You

Organizations often treat brokers as buyers' agents, but the reality is that their financial incentives typically make them sellers' agents for your insurance carrier and other health benefits vendors. Benefits consulting is a $22 billion industry, and insurance companies are the source for much of that revenue.[99] According to industry veterans, over 90 percent of the compensation models for brokers conflict with your objectives, because their income increases as overall per capita health care spending increases. In a proper model, one would expect exactly the opposite: Compensation should *decrease* as low-value spending increases. Over the last few decades of consistent health care spending increases, status quo brokers have won big while employers and their employees have lost.

Most disturbing is that brokers generally don't disclose a significant portion of their compensation. For example, insurance carriers and other vendors work to retain clients by tying broker commission and bonus programs to the total business the broker places with the carrier, not just your business. Brokers typically must clear a specific threshold of business each year to get these bonuses. *Your business is just one piece of the total, but keeping it with the same carrier can boost the broker's total compensation by 50 percent or more.* Because this compensation isn't specific to you, status quo brokers will often claim they've disclosed fees and commissions. But they are actually only disclosing your *account-specific* fees and commissions that may not even be the most significant piece of their overall compensation.

Another way insurance carriers enforce loyalty is a clause in broker contracts that let carriers drop brokers on 30-day notice. If a broker gets over half of their entire compensation from a specific carrier—a common situation that can include annuity-type compensation built up over years—you can imagine how potent that threat is. Forward-looking brokers have sent me letters from insurance carriers saying they'd be "fired" when they spoke the truth about egregious practices the carrier was inflicting on the broker's clients. This makes clear that the carriers view brokers as a quasi-employee they can fire at will. In other words, they are working for the carrier, not your organization.

Flawed Assumption #2: Insurance Carriers Want to Drive Down Costs and PPO Networks Deliver the Best Pricing

Much of pricing in health care is set as a percentage of Medicare pricing. Why? Because Medicare uses a rigorous process to develop pricing that takes into account actual hospital costs (which are often inflated, but we cover that elsewhere) and market variances. The average PPO network pricing is 2.6 times Medicare rates or, as it is often called, "260 percent of Medicare." While there are some markets where average commercial payer pricing is lower, there are many more where the number is significantly greater—as high as 1,000 percent of Medicare in some places.[100]

To get a deeper perspective, I spoke with Mike Dendy, an industry veteran with deep health care cost management experience. Dendy was previously chairman/CEO of HPS Paradigm Administrators, an independent third-party administrator (TPA) services company that manages both private- and public-sector plans. Before that, he was the head of community health system business at Memorial Hospital in Savannah, Georgia.

Dendy's company managed a large volume of claims. On average, he says they found that hospitals bill services (called gross billed charges) at about 550 percent of Medicare and that the major insurance carrier PPO network discounts are approximately 50 percent off those prices.

"It is amazing how little employers know about what they pay. I met with a Fortune 100 company that has 110,000 U.S.-based employees and asked their human resources vice president how much they were paying for health care relative to the Medicare benchmark. He had no clue and was flabbergasted when I gave him the answer. The BUCAs [Blue Cross, UnitedHealthcare, Cigna, and Aetna] hide that information, of course."

In comparison, employers who properly manage their health care spend will often pay roughly 150 percent of Medicare rates. Their logic is that the government has arrived at a price that would enable health care organizations to sustain themselves, so hospitals should be willing to limit themselves to a 50 percent premium on top of that. Some will accept 120 percent or less.

However, most employers play the PPO's discount game without question. There is a "wink, wink, nod, nod" exercise that insurance carriers and health providers go through to arrive at a baseline PPO network price, which allows carriers to say they "negotiated" a larger discount, say 52 percent. This makes it appear that the network can get you a better deal than you can on your own. Hey, I'll give you a 99 percent discount on anything if I get to choose the undiscounted price.

To add insult to injury, PPO networks charge access fees of $12-$20 per employee per month (PEPM) for what you might call the privilege of overpaying for health care services. Insurance carriers continue to insist to employers that their employees won't be able to see a doctor or be admitted to a hospital outside the PPO network relationship. This is every bit as ludicrous as it sounds. Care provider organizations are often eager to develop direct payment arrangements that are far better than typical PPO rates.

Flawed Assumption #3: Auto-Adjudication of Claims Is Always Good

Auto-adjudication is the term used to describe automatic payment of claims. Claims administrators will highlight one of three specific benefits of this system: Your employees won't be hassled with bills, it's a sign of efficiency, or it's based on sophisticated algorithms— typically all three. However, the best way to describe auto-adjudication is that you're giving another organization a blank check to withdraw money from your treasury based on minimal information that may or may not even be accurate.

Claims administrators from the largest national insurance companies to the smallest mom and pop shops essentially all follow the same process. They receive a useless Uniform Bill (UB) from a hospital as an invoice, deduct the PPO discount from the total price, then pay the claim.

Figure 9 is an anonymized UB provided to me by Dendy for $323,000. This one-page UB represents the entire invoice submitted by the hospital on this claim. Note that 322 units of laboratory— completely unspecified—are billed at $157,808. No one in their right mind would ever accept such minimal detail if they're spending their own money. And yet the claims administrator in this case was prepared to write the check if AMPS had not intervened.

Further, BUCA administrators often charge $30 to $60 per employee per month (PEPM) to pay bills using this see-nothing, know-nothing method. Pretty good gig if you can get it. Large insurance carriers typically auto-adjudicate 90 percent or more of all claims.[101] Dendy's firm intervened on behalf of a Fortune 100 company on a hospital bill for well over $2 million. Even he was shocked to learn that the claims administrator was ready to pay on the basis of the single-page UB.

It's no surprise that claims administrators often have clauses in their agreements with employers that would only fly in health care. What's surprising is that so many employers are willing to sign them. For example, contracts stipulate that claims data is proprietary and owned by the carrier, meaning you don't get to see your own claims data. Sometimes, they'll use HIPAA privacy as a smokescreen to prevent you from having your data analyzed by an outside party, an issue HIPAA effectively accommodates.

Second, claims administrators will insist on extremely limited claim audit clauses. One large company I'm aware of with more than two million claims per year had an audit clause that gave it the right to audit just 200 claims *of the administrator's choosing* and only on the carrier's premises. That's 0.01 percent of all claims for what is often a company's first or second largest expense after payroll.

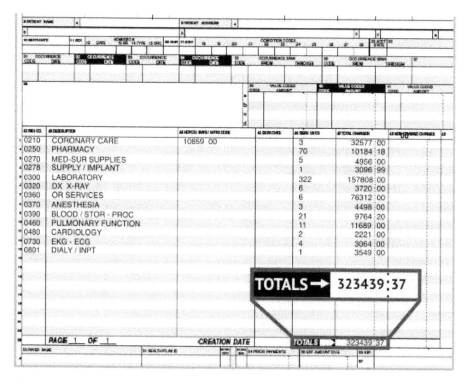

Figure 9. Actual de-identified uniform bill provided by Dendy.

Limited audit clauses often reflect an agreement between insurance carriers and health care providers. The insurance carrier will sign a PPO agreement with a hospital that, absurdly, doesn't allow the carrier itself to audit claims. The alleged reason is that it's all part of the give and take in negotiations, in which the carrier "demands" a certain discount in exchange for not auditing the claims they pay from that hospital.[102]

This dynamic is why transparent open networks featuring direct relationships between employers and hospitals have arisen (See Chapter 22 – Transparent Open Networks to learn more). By directly contracting with a health care provider, employers can secure significant savings. More direct, streamlined payment makes it valuable for high-value health care providers as well.

Key Take-aways

- Though benefits brokers sell themselves as advocates for the buyer, they are generally sales agents for insurance carriers.
- PPO networks, once a good idea, have become a core method for insurance carriers to ensure health care prices go up irrespective of underlying costs of health care services.
- Auto-adjudication of claims is rarely good.

CASE STUDY

CITY OF MILWAUKEE

John Torinus

City Slashes Health Care Costs by Improving Benefits

Because the economic pain of out-of-control medical costs is so high and Federal Government reforms are so slow, school districts, counties, and municipalities are moving on their own to find savings across the four major platforms for containing health care spending: self-insurance, consumer-driven incentives and disincentives, onsite proactive primary care, and value-based purchasing.

The City of Milwaukee, Wisconsin, with 6,500 employees, is one spectacular example. The city has held its health care costs *flat* for the last five years, stopping its previous hyper-inflationary trend of eight to nine percent annual increases. Milwaukee spent $139 million on health care in 2011 before switching over to a self-insured plan in 2012. Costs dropped to $102 million in 2012 and have stayed at about that level ever since—even in the face of six percent annual inflation for employer plans nationally over the same period.

If the old trend had continued, health costs for 2016 would have been about $200 million, double what they actually were.

Instead, the cost savings have had many additional positive ramifications: raises for county employees, no layoffs, flat employee premium contributions, better health outcomes for employees and their families, improved productivity, lower absenteeism, and less pressure to raise taxes.

Michael Brady, benefits manager, led this intelligent management approach in close collaboration with the mayor, city council, and unions. As with other enlightened group plans, there are many moving parts. Here's a sampling:

- An onsite wellness center and workplace clinic, headed by nurse practitioners, has sharply reduced hospital admissions. Onsite physical therapy was added last year. These services are free for employees and spouses.
- Relatively low deductibles (now $750 per single employee and $1,500 per family) were installed to create a consumer-friendly environment.
- Co-insurance was set at 10 percent for members who use UnitedHealthcare's Premium Provider program, which uses only doctors designated as top doctors by UnitedHealthcare. Co-insurance is 30 percent for providers outside that group. This tiered approach, aimed at improving health outcomes, is a form of value-based purchasing.
- Participants in the city's wellness program can earn $250 in a health account. Good progress has been made on hypertension and smoking (now 12 percent vs. U.S. average of 14 percent), but, as with other employers, there's not been as much traction on obesity. There have been some improvements on chronic disease management of diabetes. *
- A $200 ER copay has cut non-urgent ER visits by 300 per year.
- An intense program to reduce injuries, started in 2008, has resulted in a 70 percent drop in work hours lost to injury. The

---

* While workplace wellness programs typically have no or negative ROI (see Chapter 9-Wellness), approaches that use solid clinical evidence to address costly chronic illness and procedures without encouraging overtreatment are sometimes lumped into the same category as typical workplace wellness programs. However, they are highly different in goals, execution, and results.

program has saved $10 million per year compared to the previous trend line.

- Milwaukee now spends about $15,000 per employee per year, well below the national average and not too far off the $13,000 at the best private companies.

Government entities are not known for bold innovation, so this track record is an eye-opener, especially in a unionized environment. "The results," said Brady, "are nothing short of amazing considering changes in the city's workforce demographics and the challenging environmental hazards that city employees regularly face."

These changes have taken place at the same time that the nation as a whole has experienced much more disappointing progress from federal reforms, e.g., much higher deductibles for plans sold on ACA exchanges, double-digit premium rises for employers in many states, and a cost to the Federal government of about $5,000 per subsidized plan member per year.

Clearly, most of the meaningful reform of the economic chaos from health care in this country is coming from self-insured employers, like the City of Milwaukee.

John Torinus is chairman of Serigraph Inc., a Wisconsin-based graphics parts manufacturer, and author of "The Company That Solved Health Care."

CHAPTER 9

CRIMINAL FRAUD IS MUCH BIGGER THAN YOU THINK

"I ain't blind and I don't like what I think I see" – The Doobie Brothers, "Taking It to the Streets"

Most of us think of fraud in health care as the domain of a few bad doctors, similar to what exists in virtually any human enterprise. In reality, it adds up to a staggering $300 billion annually, roughly 10 percent of all health care spending.[103] It is also remarkably straightforward to stop, but only if claims administrators—those actually able to stop it—do so. Yet, most lack the financial incentives to do so, making only basic after-the-fact attempts that are like trying to stop fraud with a musket in an era of unmanned drones.

More alarming is that significant fraudulent gains may go to foreign actors. The world's cybercrime hotspots are all outside the United States, according to *Time*.[104] *Infoworld*[105] explained why hackers want your health care data: Among other reasons, it has a much longer shelf life than other targets like credit cards, which become useless once a consumer gets a new card. Medical and insurance information has value for years. It's bad enough that there is widespread fraud, but the fact that it is leaving the U.S. economy makes it even more of an economic drain.

Stopping fraud would be like providing the American economy with an annual $300 billion economic stimulus. Over two-plus years, that would be equivalent to the massive stimulus at the beginning of the 2008 financial crisis.

Health Insurance Carriers Are Acting Rationally

There are two key drivers of insurance carrier economics that are relevant to understanding criminal fraud (These issues were covered more thoroughly in Chapter 5 - Pressure insurance company execs face).

1. Anything that drives health care spending upward, even paying fraudulent claims, economically benefits insurance carriers and claims administrators.
2. The ACA's Medical Loss Ratio cap requires that 80 to 85 percent of premium dollars go to care, not marketing and overhead. Because fraud prevention isn't considered care, this reduces economic incentives to invest in it. Technology and other solutions that prevent fraud are just another expense that eats into this government-mandated margin cap.

Even if an employer is self-insured, there is a spillover effect because insurance carriers are generally motivated to invest in technologies and services that fuel revenue increases rather than reduce spending. In other words, there isn't a strong enough motivation to root out waste and fraud.

It's important to note how only-in-health-care dynamics open the door to large-scale fraud in the first place. Pay and chase programs (covered in Chapter 5 - Pressure insurance company execs face) are like paying a napping guard extra money to chase a criminal who just cleaned out the bank vault. According to private conversations with industry insiders, insurance companies acting as claims administrators are doing little to stop fraudulent claims. Instead, after allowing fraudulent claims to be paid with your money, they chase after the thieves, receiving 30 to 40 percent of what they recover.

The Data Problem

More fraud creates more upward premium pressure that benefits insurance carriers but takes from everyone else. The root of this is the U.S. health care system's current claims methodology, which is fraught with disconnects and a lack of transparency and control among employers, patients, providers, and insurers. In contrast, the equally large and complex financial industry has been using preventive methodologies for decades, giving consumers both security assurances and control over their credit, resulting in much lower credit card fraud rates—just 0.07 percent of total volume.[106] This means the cost of health care fraud is 14,285 percent higher than credit card fraud.

Health care has generally avoided adopting similar prevention measures, erroneously citing a billing and payment system that is too complex for it to work. Instead, employers have resorted to a reactive and largely ineffective approach to recovering money after claims have been paid. This "pay and chase" method delivers a dismal average return rate of only two to four percent—enough to say something is being done, but a drop in the bucket compared to the full magnitude of the problem.[107]

When it comes to auditing claims to identify fraud, insurance carriers have historically relied on sampling methodologies to determine whether or not the claims process is sufficiently secure. Health care claims reviews are done independently on a per-visit basis and are largely a paper-driven process. This allows fraud and waste to fall through the cracks because there is so much disparate data and no standard format for how it is analyzed and processed.

Separately, the industry has pushed toward auto-adjudicating claims as quickly as possible, a good thing if not for the lack of correspondingly robust implementation of fraud (and waste and abuse) detection and prevention technologies and processes.

"The current claims process is predicated on rapid processing of health care transactions with little real emphasis on the legitimacy and accuracy of the claims themselves," states Scott Haas, Senior Vice President of USI Insurance Services. "The Department of Labor claim processing regulations emphasize the time frame in which claim payers must either pay or deny claims. The regulations assume payers are actually diligent in assessing whether or not the claims require any form of audit or scrutiny." Such antiquated processes, disparate data, and unintended regulatory consequences create a macro-situation ripe with subjective interpretation of claims and claims data, often making the eventual reconciliation of plan coverage and payment too late. Often, this also leads to legitimate claims being denied erroneously, further adding to the frustration of everyone involved in the claims paying process. It's a costly failure for everyone.

Connecting the Data Points

Fraud only becomes visible when you connect all of the care participants and events. Here are two real-life examples I've seen.

- A woman undergoing multiple hysterectomies
- A man getting multiple circumcisions from different providers in a single week

Technically, these cases each meet all of the basic claims review and adjudication criteria (e.g., all of the fields are filled out and don't have text where numbers should be or vice versa). Therefore, they pass the sufficiency test and the claims are paid. However, it's obvious that both are fraud.

The problems that arise from not connecting the dots can be less obvious than multiple instances of one-in-a-lifetime procedures. One example is a case where four doctors provided the same service to the same patient during the same procedure. When each provider's claim is viewed independently, the claim meets sufficiency criteria and thus passes the paid claims review test. But the total amount they're charging far exceeds the total allowable amount for the contract.

Big data and technologies similar to those used for services like Visa Fraud Protection make it possible to identify, predict, and minimize fraud through advanced analytics for detecting fraud and validating claim accuracy and consistency.

Payment integrity technology is available that can analyze disparate claims data at the employer, patient, provider, and insurance carrier levels simultaneously across all health care systems. Such technology-based systems can connect a patient's behavior with the relevant physician behavior. For example, a patient who has had a hysterectomy in the past and suddenly has pregnancy-related claims should be flagged. By contrast, the financial services industry has used similar behavior patterns both at the retailer and consumer levels to identify purchases that do not fit the consumer's normal behavior since the earliest days of credit cards.

Innovative payment integrity solutions break the reactive "pay and chase" approach and could nearly eliminate fraud, making it unnecessary for employers to chase after already spent money. These types of solutions will play a critical role in reducing the exorbitant amounts of money lost to fraud and waste in the health care system every year.

Fraud and Abuse Enabling the Opioid Crisis

Without immediate intervention to break the pharmaceutical supply chain that travels from manufactures to physician subscriptions to fraudulent prescriptions to pharmacy distribution, it is impossible to estimate, at this point, the losses the United States will endure in the years ahead.

Governments and large employers that self-insure typically contract with PBMs to manage enrollment of employees and reimbursements for their pharmaceuticals, including opioids. PBMs are typically paid by the transaction or employee; it's not their money, so it's not their risk. They may strive to handle claims quickly and efficiently, but their defenses against fraud and abuse of prescription drugs are antiquated.

The shared responsibilities of the employer or government agency and the PBM create situations in which neither can see the whole picture. Criminals exploit this weakness, leading to a flood of prescription opioids on the street. The American insurance system has allowed this distribution explosion to occur, doing little to nothing to halt its growth.

Of course, willfully fraudulent claims have captured the most attention and are a growing problem. A common example is the individual who fills the same prescription, for the same phantom treatment, on the same day, at five different locations.

Generally, improper prescriptions come from two sources. One comes from fake prescriptions written by doctors for injuries that do not exist. The second is fraud from criminal organizations that use personal identities from breached databases to submit claims.

Key Take-aways

- Health care fraud is larger than entire industries such as advertising. Technology is available to solve most health care fraud as has been accomplished in financial services, but key players have disincentives to deploy the technology.
- With guards down, no industry experiences more cybercrime than health care. Most are using the equivalents of muskets in an era of unmanned drones.
- Lack of modern payment integrity software has been one of the enablers of the opioid crisis.

CHAPTER 10

ARE WORKPLACE WELLNESS PROGRAMS HAZARDOUS TO YOUR HEALTH?

"Education is the most powerful weapon which you can use to change the world." – Nelson Mandela

One area of widespread spending that typically has little benefit—and no cost savings—is workplace wellness programs. Promotion of wellness programs has been a particularly deft move by health plans to distract from their economic incentive to raise health care costs. For someone not paying attention to health care realities, it seems plausible that the fattening of America is a primary driver of increased health care spending (it's not). As the rest of the book points out, there are numerous other, much bigger cost inflation drivers even if the so-called wellness programs were effective (few are).

To start, they're usually sold on mathematically impossible ROIs and undisclosed commission models that enormously benefit brokers. This has caused Al Lewis, former workplace wellness industry proponent turned leading critic, to offer a $2 million reward to anyone who can prove that the industry has reduced employers' medical claims costs enough to cover its $8 billion annual cost.[108] So far, his money is safe.

By way of background, Lewis was a workplace wellness industry insider, called one of the founding fathers of disease management.[109] Now, he's CEO of Quizzify, a provider of employee health literacy programs, and author of several best-selling books on measuring the outcomes of employee health improvement programs, especially workplace wellness programs (check out *Surviving Workplace Wellness* and *Why Nobody Believes the Numbers*).

Promoters place workplace wellness programs among the most important advances in medical history, equivalent in impact to vaccines and antibiotics (their words).[110] Detractors call it a "scam." An entire website, www.theysaidwhat.net, is devoted to exposing its many alleged lies and misdeeds.

Obviously, it can't be both a significant advance and total scam. It's critical to know which, though, because there is a very specific distinction between workplace wellness programs and everything else in this book. Whereas everything else is an unfortunate byproduct of insuring your employees in today's status quo market, these programs are a totally optional undertaking.

Workplace wellness program fees typically cost employers $100 to $150 per employee per year. Plus, a similar amount in employee incentives to encourage usage. Plus, lost work time to participate in screening programs and complete health risk assessments. Plus, administrative time to ensure compliance with relevant laws and regulations. Add these up and you start to see that the total costs are much more than just vendor fees. All this to generate great employee dissatisfaction, judging by the fact that a 2016 *Slate* article entitled "Workplace Wellness is a Sham" generated more shares than any other *Slate* article on either health care or the workplace that year.[111]

Lewis advocates a much simpler approach to preventive care: regular screenings based on well-established clinical guidelines developed by the U.S. Preventive Services Task Force (USPSTF), an independent, volunteer panel of national experts in prevention and evidence-based medicine.[112] To balance the harms of over-screening, misdiagnosis, and over-treatment against the benefits of early detection, the USPSTF guidelines recommend far fewer blood screenings, far less frequently than most vendors advocate. These guidelines are easily accessible through the Choosing Wisely initiative, a partnership between the American Board of Internal Medicine Foundation and *Consumer Reports* that seeks to advance a national dialogue on avoiding wasteful or unnecessary medical tests, treatments, and procedures.[113]

Promoters Undercut Their Own Data

Tellingly, promoters' own data consistently and convincingly undermine their claims, which is easily shown using facts and basic arithmetic. Here are some examples to support this thesis—keep in mind that we're using what the industry says about itself.

1. A national leading workplace wellness program promoter's own conclusions and assertions have shown that a perfect workplace wellness program targeting cardiac care would have a negative ROI of $100 per employee per year.
2. An analysis in *Health Affairs* of Connecticut's workplace wellness program concluded that it increased costs. The state justified it by saying it increased the number of checkups, even though the U.S. Preventive Services Task Force Guidelines and the *Journal of the American Medical Association* have concluded that checkups don't improve health and are more likely to find problems that don't exist.
3. The guidebook of the wellness industry's trade association, the Health Enhancement Research Organization, shows that workplace wellness programs don't generate positive ROI.
4. The industry's trade publication has published articles that conclude 90 to 95 percent of workplace wellness programs have no impact and that only poorly-designed clinical studies on programs show strong ROI; one editor concluded "Who cares about an ROI anyway?"
5. The data submitted by winners of the industry's top Koop award—which is selected by wellness industry executives—over the last couple of years show that they didn't save money; in some cases, health actually deteriorated.

These are just a few examples of many I could have selected. If you want to dive deeper, Appendix F has more detailed summaries for each.

The Bottom Line

These are just a few examples of many I could have selected. If you want to dive deeper, Appendix F has more detailed summaries for each.

Money spent on workplace wellness programs—upwards of $100 to $150 per employee per year just for the vendor fees— is wasted. And this doesn't include all the peripheral tangible and intangible costs, like time spent engaging in the programs. Further, the fees cover only the administrative medical expenses, not the expenses submitted via claims forms. Superfluous annual checkups urged by vendors probably double that figure. Employee incentives to get them to use programs likely double it again.

The fastest way to create a reasonable ROI is to reduce screening frequencies to follow established, age-appropriate, USPSTF guidelines. Not only will you avoid the expense of well- ness programs, but you'll also avoid potentially harming your employees. Based on the data in this book alone, that would be a significant improvement over what is happening now.

Another possibility would be to explore the proposed 401W Savings Plan, which aligns incentives between employers and employees to work toward long-term health maintenance, while saving employers money and quite literally giving people financial responsibility for taking care of themselves.[114] It also increases employee retention, as well as program satisfaction.

Sound good so far? If you need one more reason to look into the 401W Savings Plan, here it is. As most people in the industry know, Al Lewis is the Mikey of wellness. He hates everything. But he likes this a lot.[115]

Yes, Virginia, There Are Workplace Wellness Programs That Work

Like ABC's Wide World of Sports, we've spanned the globe looking for workplace wellness programs that work. We've found three.

First is Cummins, a diesel engine manufacturer with 55,000 employees. When *Fortune*, went looking for the best, this was the one they found.[116] After years of trying to "preach the gospel" of wellness with conventional screenings, Cummins realized it wasn't working. So, they rebooted a new model with a "continuum" of services that employees could select from to reach their goals. Plus, much of what Cummins does is environmental—such as workplace design—so there is no need for employees to "opt in." Well-being comes to them.

For those who want to adopt a healthier lifestyle, Cummins offers many opt-in opportunities. This is in sharp contrast to conventional programs that try to make employees healthy whether they want it or not. No wonder they consistently make the Fortune list of the 100 best places to work.

Next, *Workforce* magazine highlighted the Hilliard County (OH) Schools.[117] Their wellness leader, Debbie Youngblood, had the insight that, for example, you can't teach employees to eat less sugar if they don't know where that sugar is hidden in the ingredients labels.

"It always surprises me," says Ms. Youngblood, "that we expect people to know how to achieve overall well-being. [Yet] we've given them very little opportunity to know, understand, and practice the things that might be beneficial."

For a third example, we turned to the very same Al Lewis who basically finds fault in everything workplace wellness and challenged him to come up with one. Surely, in all his travels, he had found a single program—just one—that worked. He thought for a minute and then said, "Wait a sec! The one I'm in, Boston College's, is great. They actually screen me according to guidelines. I mean, that shouldn't win them a Nobel Prize, but in this industry, it does.

"Plus, when I go in for my screen—every three years, just like the guidelines say—I'm always trying to find fault, but, instead, I am amazed at how good the guidance is. Totally up to date on carbs and fat, no telling me to get a PSA test or other inappropriate interventions, and knowledgeable staff. And no wonder. They get their program from Harvard Pilgrim Health Care, the top-ranked health plan in the country basically every year, according to the National Committee for Quality Assurance."

Key Take-aways

- By the wellness industry's own figures, there is a negative ROI to the vast majority of wellness programs.
- Most wellness programs increase the risk of overtreatment, putting employees' well-being at risk.
- Wellness programs are optional and money is better spent on what truly drives health and well-being, such as value-based primary care.

Part III

Doing It Right

*A*s we say on the Health Rosetta website, "Health care is already *fixed. Join us to replicate the fixes."*

Fortunately, whether private or public sector, rural or urban, small or large, employers in virtually every corner of the country have proven that they can reduce spending by 20 percent or more compared to average employers while significantly improving benefits programs. In this part of the book, we lay out the most important building blocks and mindsets. We explore how, together, a transparent benefits advisor or consultant relationship and an independent claims administrator is often the best path to capturing the greatest value from your health dollars.

"Employees are our greatest asset" is a common expression, yet many companies don't operate that way. In highly competitive markets, leading employers are creating advantage through innovative benefits plans built around high-value components that are often ignored or underutilized, such as primary care and mental health services. This section gives you the new mindset and tools to do this reset.

CHAPTER 11

YOU RUN A HEALTH CARE BUSINESS WHETHER YOU LIKE IT OR NOT

Here's How to Make It Thrive

"GM is a health and benefits company with an auto company attached." – Warren Buffett

GM spends more on health care than steel, just as Starbucks spends more on health care than coffee beans.

For most companies, health care is the second largest expense after payroll. This puts you in the health care business.

So, how's your health care business doing?

When the COO of a large private equity fund's health care benefits purchasing group sits down with the CEO of a newly acquired company, say a manufacturer, that's the first question he asks. Naturally, the CEO will look puzzled. The COO will then show that the company has, for example, 4,200 members enrolled in their health plan and spends the typical $10,000 per year per member for health care. He then rephrases the question: "How's your $42 million health care business?"

"That's when the light bulb goes on," said the COO.

A Shift in Mindset

As we have seen, most organizations don't apply the same level of care to their health care spending that they do to other large expenditures. Estimates of fraud, waste, and abuse in health care range from a low of 30 percent (Institute of Medicine) to over 50 percent (PwC) but are little known among employers.[118] Note that these are the same companies that often manage other major budget items down to the hundredths of a percent, yet regularly accept 5 to 20 percent annual health care cost increases. In most cases, they have an overburdened, outgunned HR leader who is overseeing the health care spend with little or no analytic capabilities.

The reality is most companies wouldn't hire their present benefits leader to run a multimillion dollar business unit or product. Then why are they running a multimillion dollar benefits spend?

So, what's different about employers who are winning the battle to slay the health care cost beast? It's all about mindset. It's about waking up to the understanding that improving the value of health benefits is the best way to improve the well-being of their employees while boosting the company's bottom line—and then committing to that path.

"In virtually every case," the COO said, "employers who have seen the light and taken action see their health care costs flatten or decline a bit, while other employers continue to face ever-increasing care costs. Soon they're spending 20 percent less on health benefits per capita. Eventually, the most successful are spending 40-55 percent less. Plus, the financial and other advantages of waking up compound over time. As each year passes, the gap between wide-awake employers and those accepting the status quo grows."

As I've traveled to every corner of the country, I've seen wide-awake employers—large and small, rural and urban, public and private sector—who refuse to buy into what I believe has become the biggest lie in health care: that health care costs can't be controlled.

However, it's not just about costs. We've long heard leaders state that employees are their most important asset. These wide-awake employers, from IBM to a small poultry processor in rural Wisconsin, have shifted their benefits mindset to match. Instead of looking at health benefits as a soft HR benefit, they now see them as investments in health and well-being that are strategic inputs to their supply chain and P&L. They manage health benefits programs accordingly.

Fair Trade for Health Care

In choosing care provider partners, wide-awake employers understand that the well-being of caregivers has a direct impact on the care of their employees. It's enlightened self-interest to make sure that physicians and other clinical staff are not abused by administrators, working conditions, compensation models, unbridled profit incentives, and other challenges that are, sadly, very common. If the people running the show exhibit disdain for their own staff, how do you think they'll treat yours?

If you've ever bought Fair Trade coffee, you've probably done so in a deliberate effort to say no to products produced by child or slave labor, or whose owners run roughshod over the environment. I'm proposing that you likewise insist that health care organizations exhibit fair and ethical treatment of clinicians and patients before you become one of the latter. Here's what Fair Trade for health care should include.

- *Transparent prices.* Upfront pricing should be readily available without having to subscribe to a special service. Hospitals, physicians, and labs should have continued freedom to set their own prices, but predatory pricing, with a different rate for each person, is out of the question.
- *Bundled prices.* Imagine buying a car and getting a bill for the transmission six months later. You'd be livid, yet

this sort of thing happens all the time in the health care industry. A transparent price must include the full bundle of services that wrap around it. This is the norm for the transparent open network we discuss later in this book. While not every area of health care will fit into a bundle, it's broader than you might imagine. For example, the University of Oklahoma's Harold Hamm Diabetes Center has an all-in bundle for diabetes management at different severity levels.

- *A culture of safety.* Given that preventable medical errors are a leading cause of death in America and bring untold misery to millions of patients every year, one of the best ways to identify a safe hospital is to ask nurses if they would want a family member to receive care in their facility and, if so, by which unit-level team. In fact, the Joint Commission (the U.S. accrediting body for hospitals) strongly recommends that hospitals measure safety culture, and most do, but this information is not shared with the public. Leapfrog Group safety scores are a great source for assessing this.

- *Staff treatment*: Physicians and nurses are suffering from record levels of suicide and burnout. To think this doesn't affect the quality of care they provide is naive. Research shows that patient outcomes are correlated with how a hospital treats its clinical staff.[119]

- *Ethics-based organizations.* There must be a focus on patient-reported outcomes. That is, outcomes like living without pain or playing a sport—not just having a successful surgery, especially if it would have been better to avoid going into the OR in the first place. Virginia Mason Hospital & Medical Center in Seattle, a forward-looking organization, has been candid in admitting that, at one time, 90 percent of its spinal procedures were of no help.[120]

While some worry about rationing care, the volume-driven reimbursement system has always rationed choices by pushing us toward costly, invasive treatment options. Top-performing, value-based primary care organizations tell us that patients virtually always choose the least invasive treatment option first—but only if they're told about sound alternatives to expensive and overused treatments and tests. Equipping patients to become active partners in their own care is the sign of an ethical organization. So are ethical business practices, which don't include intimidating doctors into relationships with a local hospital, an unfortunate and common practice.

- *Data liquidity*. Care teams do their best work when they have the most complete view of a patient's health status. Anything less comes with an increased risk of harm. Likewise, your employees should have easy access to their own information in a secure, patient-controlled data repository—including the right to contribute their own data or take it elsewhere.

Two Stories

In the 2000s, IBM made a mindset shift about employee welfare and decided to integrate its health services. According to Paul Grundy, MD, and Martin Sepulveda, MD—the physicians who led these efforts—the company realized they were competing against giants like WiPro and Infosys from India, which have much lower cost structures. IBM would have to tackle the cost side of the equation, but they also saw that they could gain a strategic advantage if they had much higher-performing teams. Accordingly, they put a particular focus on the fitness, productivity, and resilience of their workforce.

Sepulveda described to me their revelation that indiscriminate provision of health care services—absent efforts to help people understand how to use those services—leads to voracious appetites from both patients and providers for services that add little value but add a lot of cost to the individual, company, and society.

It dawned on him that if they were going to develop a worldwide health care strategy, they would have to build on universal values. People everywhere value health, access, receiving health care, and relationships in health care. It was striking to Sepulveda how important the relationship is between the person receiving care and the person delivering the care. What people understand and what they are willing to do is greatly influenced by that interaction. The ideal setting, he saw, is a full-function primary care setting that includes behavioral health and health coaching.

The challenge for a global leader like IBM was to develop a strategy that would work in vastly different environments: in rapid-growth countries with poor infrastructure, in a socialized country like France, and in a private insurance country like the United States. They decided that, all other things being equal, they would put a third of their health care chips on prevention, a third on primary care, and a third on employee engagement with (and accountability for) their own health and with the health care system. The result is that IBM has built itself a competitive advantage with a lower cost structure and a higher-performing workforce.

On the other end of the spectrum with a very similar success story is Brakebush, a small poultry processor in rural Wisconsin with 1,700 employees, many of whom are at high risk for injuries due to the nature of their job. For Brakebush, the wake-up call was a realization that they were pouring major resources into one of health care's most notorious money pits: musculoskeletal (MSK) procedures based on no scientific evidence, which, in most cases, provide less value than physical therapy (PT).[121]

They took a multipronged approach to eliminating the waste, including allocating resources to address and mitigate physical risks in their plants, hiring an onsite PT specialist to provide MSK care in a value-based fee model, and creating a new health care coordinator position to help employees navigate the health system. Brakebush now incentivizes employees who do need surgery to use designated centers of excellence for procedures that come with an upfront bundled price and warranty. They also use price transparency tools, a health care concierge, and health coaching. And in 2016, the company opened a health center that provides primary care, personal training, and a gym—at no cost to employees.

Sounds like a big investment, right? Yet Brakebush paid less for health care in 2016 than it did in 2014. It now spends 50 percent less than average for companies their size on MSK disorders, saving $1 million a year on just this one area.

What to Look for in a Health Plan Administrator

Obviously, you can't ask most HR benefits directors to pull off this kind of culture change. What you need is a sophisticated health administrator, analogous to the person who's administering your 401(k). This is someone whose skills and experience are commensurate with the magnitude of your investment in health benefits and the level of fiduciary responsibility it carries.

You want a person who is both numbers and people savvy, who understands the inner workings of a health plan, and who can bring real solutions to bear in a way that aligns the incentives of all parties. And then you want to give him or her the clout to get the job done with the respect and support of the C-suite. Depending on the size of your organization, this may be an outside advisor. This person must also be empowered with financial and other performance incentives that align with lowering costs and improving outcomes.

In short, you need someone able to run a complex supply chain. Here are some characteristics to look for.

- Outstanding finance skills with a focus on accuracy in forecasting and communicating stories through numbers
- Keen understanding that many types of cost-shifting to employees add financial stress that negatively impacts employee well-being and productivity
- Relentless focus on rooting out status quo health care industry practices designed to redistribute wealth and profits from you to them, including disclosure of commissions and fees, such as hidden bonus structures like insurance carrier overrides paid to benefits brokers
- Ability to understand and carry out ERISA and other fiduciary responsibilities for administering a high-performance health plan
- Insight into the moral impact and financial objectives of change and genuine concern for employees and their families
- Good communication skills
- Strong analytic, statistical, and actuarial skills to evaluate ROI in an industry that plays fast and loose with both promises and numbers
- Indefatigable learning, seeking proven solutions from any corner of the country / industry and innovative ideas that will disrupt the status quo
- Intimacy with the current state of affairs relating to health insurance and health care (i.e., not reliant on information spoon-fed by brokers)
- Ability to build consensus among influential peers, typically other employers and ideally those with large numbers of employees. The greatest leverage, by far, is in numbers.

Key Take-aways

- Match the talent and resources to the magnitude of the health benefits task.
- Expect and demand the same level of quality, safety, and transparency in health care that you do in all other areas of your organization.

- From small manufacturers in rural America to large, urban multinationals, it's entirely possible to expect better benefits for the same or less money every year – not unlike every other item in your budget. There's no need to accept the norm of getting less and paying more.

CHAPTER 12

HOW TO PICK A BENEFITS CONSULTANT

David Contorno

Recently, a Blue Cross health plan offered their brokers a $50,000 reward for switching self-insured clients back to more lucrative, fully-insured plans. In sectors like financial services, that kind of undisclosed conflict could land a person in jail. In health care, however, such clear conflicts of interest are common and considered "business as usual."

For most companies, health care spending is one of the largest expenses on the P&L, often ranking in the top two or three. However, few business leaders give it any more time and attention than they do, say travel or entertainment expenses. Furthermore, some still leave benefits decisions up to the HR department, a seemingly well-intentioned strategy. However, taking an HR-knows-best approach is contrary to the organization's (and often employees') best interests. While HR is critical when it comes to rolling out, administering, and the required employee social counseling of your health plan, financial decisions are best left to officers with an innate ability to negotiate the highly complex.

HR professionals typically fall into one of three categories: coordinator (admin), generalist (social worker), manager (expert). Ruling out the first two as negotiators, expecting your

117

HR manager to deftly navigate a financial win while simultaneously managing recruiting, compliance, compensation, and the entire HRIS system, is akin to finding a unicorn in your driveway tonight. If your broker works closely with HR, and takes your CFO golfing twice a year, he or she is likely paying for the trip with a $50,000 carrier incentive.

Knowing how to select a benefits advisor or consultant* who has the right skill sets and integrity in an industry that is often deliberately opaque can make all the difference in delivering true value to your employees. If you'd like an example of client-first consulting, see the Appendix I "Decoding a fully insured renewal", written by Wes Spencer, an advisor from Michigan.

How We Got Here

Some historical context is important here. In the '70s and '80s, when provider networks were first created, it was generally perceived as a very good thing for the industry and overall health care costs. For the first time, an insurance carrier could negotiate lower, predetermined prices and, in return, drive patients to the providers that agreed to accept these prices.

This allowed carriers to differentiate their networks through the discounts they negotiated with providers, a marketing message that continues to this day. Further, it allowed them to grow market share and, at least in some areas, drive health care financing costs. One thing that didn't change was paying brokers a commission on the premiums of the policies they sell, which dates back to the first life insurance policies sold in the 1800s.

Fast forward to 2010 and the passage of the Affordable Care Act (ACA). One provision, known as the Medical Loss Ratio

---

The more common term is broker and there are certainly some excellent brokers that do more than connect insurance carriers and employers, but the terms advisor or consultant speak to the need for a trusted partner who works closely with you to provide a broader range of services and better alignment with your interests. It reflects common usage in the self-insured market, but you should look more deeply than what someone calls themselves.

requirement, was created with good intentions. The premise was that requiring carriers to spend a minimum of 80 to 85 percent of premiums (depending on plan type and employer size) on paying medical claims would prevent them from being overly profitable and would help control costs. It hasn't turned out this way for several reasons. First, after paying medical claims, broker commissions, and normal administrative costs, carriers weren't making an unreasonable profit in the first place. In fact, it is a far smaller percentage of revenue than most businesses would be able to survive on, albeit a small percentage of a VERY large number.

Second, because profit is now tied to a percentage of premium, which is a function of underlying medical costs, the carrier now has an increased financial incentive to ignore rising costs, so long as their costs don't rise any faster than those of their competitors. This certainly existed before 2010, but the ACA turbo-charged the dynamic. The common impression that insurance carriers' large networks and client pools gives them greater leverage in negotiating prices with providers could not be further from the truth. The more patients a hospital system treats from any particular carrier, the more leverage *the hospital system* has to increase fees. And employers unwittingly empower the provider's abuse by threatening to leave the carrier if they are unable to come to an agreement to keep that large local health care system in the network, even if it performs poorly.

For many years, all but the very largest employers have been fully invested in this arrangement. Brokers were paid a percentage of premium, employers deferred the entire responsibility for controlling costs to the insurance carrier, individuals consumed whatever care their clinician advised, and everybody was supposedly happy. But as underlying medical costs have gone up, the only winners are the insurance company, care providers (especially hospitals), drug manufacturers, pharmacy benefits managers, and, of course, brokers.

A Broken Process

Here's what typically happens every year for those employ-ers that are fully-insured. We will talk about how this works for self-insured organizations shortly.

Around 60 days prior to the contract renewal date, your bro-ker gets a renewal offer from the current carrier that has VERY lit-tle information, explaining the proposed new premiums, which they can now use to shop around the market for a better offer. Note that this market is now tiny. There were 23 national health insurance carriers in 1990; there are now just four.

Let's pause for a moment to consider that the broker often gets no information at all if you have fewer than 100 employees.

Even larger employers do not get full transparency, let alone proactive tools to address the underlying medical costs suppos-edly driving the new, higher rates. If your carrier released more data on your spending, their competitors would be able to "cherry pick" the money-making groups, weeding out the minority that loses them money every year.

Let's assume you are in that minority of money-losing cli-ents. Your carrier has to make you a renewal offer by law. So why wouldn't they just make that offer astronomically high? Because an offer with too large an increase scares off all the other carriers, making it less likely they can get rid of you as a customer, and brings them bad PR to boot.

Playing the Competition

Generally, carriers that want to win your business try to price their offer as high as they can while staying low enough to motivate you to move. That motivation used to be around a 10 percent premium delta, but with costs so high and employers accepting that switching carriers is just part of the game, the delta has shrunk significantly in recent years. Say your initial renewal offer from your current carrier is 18 percent. One of the other carriers believes you'll move for a six percent spread, so they offer a 12 percent increase over your current rates.

If your broker is loyal to your current carrier—and they usually are, because the more clients they have with one carrier, the bigger their bonus income—he or she will share that 12 percent offer with them. Naturally, that carrier doesn't have to try as hard because they already have your business, so maybe they match the new offer or come in at one percent above or below it.

Some brokers stop right there. They've shown their "value" by reducing the renewal rate by six percent, which can equal hundreds of thousands of dollars in some cases! Plus, you get to keep your current plan and stay with the "preferred" carrier in your state. Oh, and your broker gets a 12 percent pay raise for his efforts—and possibly additional bonus compensation.

Some brokers will send the matching offer back to the other carrier, pitting the two against each other and maybe squeezing out another few points. Either way, your rates are no longer about the cost of your employees' care. They are now about the carriers charging as much as they can while keeping the customers they want. Note that, in the unlikely event your broker was able to save you 20 percent on your premiums, he or she would also take a 20 percent haircut.

The Bottom Line

Once the bottom-line number is reached, if the increase is still more than your budget can handle, the broker will then offer alternative options that inevitably reduce benefits. One impact of reduced benefits has been a dramatic increase in employee out-of-pocket (OOP) costs in recent years, which has made the average worker afraid to even use their plan. Of course, this causes a delay in care until the person is much sicker, creating both a larger claim down the road and additional upward pressure on future rates (not to mention often leaving the employee in a catastrophic financial situation).

One last trick to beware of: Brokers love to wait until the last minute to meet with you to review your upcoming plan renewal. Why? It may be that they are proverbially "fat and happy" and see no need to cater to your needs or perspective. It may be that they have bad news to deliver and prefer to delay tough conversations. Most likely, they feel it will reduce your ability to talk with other brokers and perhaps make a change.

Why do so many brokers support this system? For one thing, it's all they've known. The average age of the typical broker is well into their 50s. For another, as premiums go up, so do their commissions, and carriers offer large bonuses to brokers when they both sell new business and keep the old business where it is. With few exceptions, most states allow for very large "incentive" compensation to brokers. This can mean lavish trips and, more important, as much as a 67 percent increase in pay over the percent paid for the same business to a less loyal broker.[122]

Unless your organization has fewer than 20 people in your health plan, you'd more than likely get great benefits from being self-insured. If your broker/consultant doesn't have that expertise, you are being steered to a plan that benefits the carrier and broker more than you. Many advisors do have that expertise, so be careful about being a guinea pig if the broker has little experience to draw upon.

The No Shop Offer

"David Contorno, because you are such a great partner, we have an amazing offer for our mutual client! If you renew this client without shopping the market, we will come in with an amazingly low renewal AND you will qualify for a $2,500 early renewal bonus! Is this something you would be interested in receiving?"

This is an actual email I, as a benefits consultant, received from a large, well known carrier. It's a tempting offer...I feel like I am in an infomercial of fast talk and supposed deals where all I have to do is act quick and I will get a better deal for me and my client! In my head, I hear the ShamWow guy yelling "If you order in the next 24 hours, we will give you the best deal of your life! But wait, there's more! Act NOW, and we will double your order to include an embedded wellness program, and free telemedicine! But that's not all! We will pay you an additional $2,500! But you must act now!"

Please allow me to translate above... "We at carrier ABC are making so much money on this case, we don't want anyone else possibly exposing that or stealing this nugget of gold from our membership base. Since your expectations of renewals are so low, we don't actually have to price this fairly, all we have to do is come out with a better than expected increase and everyone wins!"

I have to admit, I was seduced by this offer for a long time. I can recall one case, where I was working with my "preferred" carrier at the time, on an existing client. The carrier came to me about 75 days before renewal with a no shop conversation. I asked them where they would be at, absolute bottom line best number, if I agreed to not shop it. They said 5% increase. That seemed extremely reasonable in light of the increases I was getting right around the time when the ACA was being rolled out. When I committed, on my client's behalf (without talking to them) to the offer, I was unaware that the client was already talking to another broker and that broker was out shopping the market. So, I had to back track on my "no-shop" promise. The carrier did not like this. The sales manager, to this day, still appears to hold animosity towards me over this case. But here was the outcome...when I was backed into a corner, and had to shop it, the "preferred" carrier of the other broker was coming in exactly in line with the pre-renewal rates. So, I had to push back on the current carrier, completely usurping my promise not to shop it. At the end of the day, we kept the current carrier and plans, but instead of a 5% increase, we wound up at a 5% decrease... what a great no-shop offer!

Now, if any of you reading this know me, you know this is not a good approach to managing healthcare costs. This is what we as an industry have been doing for decades, and I think the trend speaks for itself. Is a 5% decrease better than a 5% increase? Absolutely.... but when we got this client into a proper self-insured plan about 2 years ago, their costs went down by 41%! And at the same time we reduced out of pocket exposure for most procedures and services to zero for the employee!

The Self-Insured Market

How does this translate to the self-insured market? Most consultants (although not all) who support self-insured plans are far more sophisticated than the brokers profiled earlier. If they're not, self-insured plans can be a financial disaster of epic proportions. Let's assume this is not the case. A consultant in this space needs to know (1) how to set up a plan and build it out component by component and (2) how to put protections in place for your company to ensure your liability is no greater than you can financially stomach. After all, now you're the insurer and "no lifetime cap" can be a scary proposition. However, a properly set up self-insured plan actually gives you far more control of costs than a fully-insured plan. With stop-loss protection, it also lets you tailor your level of comfort with risk.

Here are the main components of high-performing self-insured plans.

- The third-party administrator (TPA) that is responsible for paying claims (with your money) according to the specifications you set up and the supporting plan documents
- The network (usually "rented" from a large carrier) that provides "discounts" off billed charges
- Balance billing protection. Employers have a duty under ERISA to only pay fair and reasonable charges. After that price is determined and paid, some providers will pursue an employee to try to get additional payment. A proper plan protects employees against this; in extreme cases, it can include legal services for the employee.
- A pharmacy manager to handle the pharmacy network

- Pricing contracts
- Stop-loss protection to pay for large claims

So now you are self-insured and are seeing a level of claims and spending detail you've never seen before. Yet costs are still going up each year at a similar rate, or maybe you saved some money the first couple of years. But now what? This is where the rubber meets the road for the more advanced consultant.

A common first misstep to lower costs is workplace wellness programs. As we saw in Are Workplace Wellness Programs Hazardous to Your Health? at best, only a tiny percentage of such programs have a real ROI. At worst, they can cost a bunch more money while irritating and potentially actually harming your employees. At least, in the self-insured environment, you have access to data that can point you toward risk factors to focus on (or scuttle the entire program). But the initial excitement and enthusiasm over data access and your fancy new workplace wellness program quickly dies. Seventy-two percent of companies have these programs and, I assure you, Seventy-two percent of companies are not happy with their health care spending trends.

Instead, a progressive consultant brings you a multiyear health care plan designed to lower the price and use of overtreatment, which harms employees financially and potentially medically. The plan is built on a proven approach to lowering the actual cost of care for ALL employees, whether they are healthy or not, and will generally reflect the following:

- Serious thought for ERISA fiduciary responsibility
- An emphasis on value-based primary care
- An emphasis on the highest-cost outlier patients
- Transparent open networks/reference-based pricing (i.e., ways to know the actual prices you'll pay for services)
- Transparent pharmacy benefits
- Data proficiency

The plan will also include payment arrangements with providers and, importantly, complete disclosure of the consultant's sources of compensation.

Value Counts More Than Fees

However, none of this can take place if your company makes one very common mistake: selecting a consultant at the same time you select your plans and other benefits for the upcoming year. A forward-looking consultant will help you see these as two distinct decisions that should be made at separate times.

As you can see, the actual "insurance" is a smaller and smaller piece of what the nontraditional benefits consultant brings to the table. In the self-insured model, stop-loss is the only insurance policy purchased, generally accounting for less than 20 percent of overall costs. Your consultant should be able to provide you with all the information you need to identify the best renewal options for noninsurance administrative functions and, critically, the right strategies to positively impact both the cost and quality of your employees' care over the long term.

You don't necessarily want to pick your consultant based on how low their fee is. (Fees are usually a small percentage, in the low single digits, of your total health care spend, which doesn't speak to their true value.) This is how most businesses make that decision, and we all know how well that's been working. A truly innovative consultant will be willing to put some of their compensation at risk, based on performance, and turn the commission conundrum described earlier on its head. Imagine paying your consultant more based on money actually saved! Now that's aligning incentives.

While no one expects an organization leader to be an expert in all these areas, you should be generally aware enough to ensure that the people trusted with handling one of your largest expenses are. Pick your benefits advisor with greater care than you would pick a 401-k advisor. After all, not only is there the same ERISA fiduciary liability as 401-k plans, a status quo plan can subject your employees to unnecessary medical harm.

One way you can judge a consultant's skill, integrity, and expertise is whether they're certified by the Health Rosetta. Certification requires transparency, expertise in key areas and strategies, and adherence to valid cost and outcome measurement models. Many seasoned, high integrity professionals have already received this qualification. Learn more at healthrosetta. org/employers.

David Contorno is a nationally recognized speaker, author and founder of E Powered Benefits which helps employers and brokers to lower costs and improve outcomes.

Key Take-aways

- If your health care costs have increased over the course of the last 5 years, there is a good chance you need a new advisor. [See Chapter 12 for more.]
- Separate the annual benefits process from the benefits advisor decision by as much time as possible.
- Beware of brokers unwilling to align your financial interests with theirs. At the same time, value counts more than fees, so avoid being penny wise and pound foolish.

CASE STUDY
LANGDALE INDUSTRIES

Brian Klepper

A Rural Wood Products Company in a One-Hospital Town Saves Hugely While Ensuring Great Care

Large American businesses with tens or hundreds of thousands of employees have recruited high-profile benefits professionals to orchestrate sophisticated campaigns focused on the health of employees and their families, and on the cost-effectiveness of their programs. Even so, few large firms provide comprehensive, quality benefits at a cost that remains consistently below national averages.

For midsized businesses—firms with 100 to 5,000 employees—the task is significantly more difficult without the right people and focus. Health benefits managers in these companies have far fewer resources, typically work alone without the benefit of a large staff, and are often overwhelmed by the complexity of their tasks. As a result, they often default to whatever their broker and health plan suggest.

But, some excel. For them, managing the many different issues—chronic disease, patient engagement, physician self-referrals, specialist and inpatient overutilization, pharmacy man-agement—is a discipline. Barbara Barrett is one of them.

Barrett is director of benefits at TLC Benefit Solutions, Inc., the benefits management arm of Valdosta, Georgia-based Lang-dale Industries, Inc., a small conglomerate of 24 firms and 1,000 employees. Langdale is engaged primarily in producing wood products for the building construction industry, but is also in car dealerships, energy, and other industries.

Valdosta is rural, which puts health benefits programs at a disadvantage. Often, as in this case, there is only one hospital nearby, which means little if any cost competition. Compared with those living in urban areas, rural Georgians are more likely to be less healthy and suffer from heart disease, obesity, diabetes, and cancer. So, the situation is far from ideal.

And yet, from 2000, when Barrett assumed responsibility for the management of Langdale's employee health benefits, to 2009, per employee costs rose from $5,400/year to $6,072/year. That's an average increase of 1.31 percent per year, compared to an average annual increase of 8.83 percent for comparably-sized firms nationally.[123] To put this in context, average firms spent $29 million more than Langdale from 2000 to 2009 to provide the same kind of coverage. Langdale's savings were $29,000 per employee—all without reducing the quality of benefits or trans-ferring the cost burden to employees.

Langdale Industries

Actual Premium* vs. US Trend and Cumulative Savings					
Year	US Trend**	Langdale (US Trend)	Langdale Actual***	Diff.	Diff. x 1,000 Eligible Emps.
2000		$5,400	$5,400		
2001	11.2%	$6,005	$5,741	$534	$534,060
2002	14.0%	$6,845	$5,542	$1,303	$1,303,065

2003	12.6%	$7,708	$5,615	$2,093	$2,093,989
2004	10.1%	$8,487	$5,689	$2,798	$2,798,941
2005	9.7%	$9,310	$5,763	$3,547	$3,547,612
2006	5.0%	$9,775	$5,839	$3,937	$3,937,601
2007	5.7%	$10,332	$5,915	$4,417	$4,417,301
2008	6.0%	$10,952	$5,993	$4,960	$4,960,756
2009	5.6%	$11,566	$6,071	$5,495	$5,495,583
Cumulative Savings $29,082,906					

*For Medical, Dental, and Pharmacy
**Source - Kaiser/HRET 2009 Employer Health Benefits Annual Survey
***Trended at an average of 1.31 percent between 2000 and 2009

So how did Barrett approach the problem? Here are a few of her strategies.

- Langdale set up TLC Benefit Solutions, a HIPAA-compliant firm that administers and processes the company's medical, dental, and drug claims. This allows Barrett to more directly track, manage, and control claim overpayments, waste, and abuse.
- It also gives her immediate access to quality and cost data on doctors, hospitals, and other vendors. Supplementing this data with external information, like Medicare cost reports for hospitals in the region, has allowed her to identify physicians and hospital services that provide low or high value. She has created incentives that steer individuals to high-value physicians and services and away from low-value ones. When necessary complex services are not available locally or have low quality or value, she shops the larger region, often sending patients to higher value centers as far away as Atlanta, three and a half hours by car.

- Barrett analyzes claims data to identify which individuals have chronic disease and which are likely to have a major acute event over the next year. Individuals with chronic diseases are directed into the company's evidence-based, opt-out disease management and prevention program. Individuals with acute care needs are connected with a physician for immediate intervention.
- Langdale provides employees and their families with confidential health advocate services that explain and encourage use of the company's benefits programs, again using targeted incentives to reward those who enter the programs and meet evidence-based targets.

These are just a few of Barrett's initiatives in group health, but her responsibilities also extend to life insurance, flex plan, supplemental benefits, retirement plan, workers' compensation, liability, and risk insurance. The results for Langdale in these areas include lower than average absenteeism, disability costs, and turnover costs.

The point isn't that you should just do what Barrett and Langdale have done. The point is that they've been proactive, endlessly innovative, and aggressive about managing the process. This attitude and rigor has paid off through tremendous savings, yes, but it has also produced a corporate culture that demonstrates the value of Langdale's employees and community. Employees and their families are healthier as a result and are more productive at work. This has borne unexpected fruit: The industries Langdale is in were hit particularly hard by the recession, and the benefits savings from Barrett's efforts helped save jobs.

Barbara Barrett and many others like her on the front line are virtually unknown in health care. Most often, their achievements go unnoticed beyond the executive offices. But they manage the health care and costs of populations in a way that all groups can be managed.

Editor's note: We checked in with Barbara recently and found that, even in the face of new challenges, such as extreme jumps in drug prices, Langdale continues to succeed where others have failed to carefully manage health costs.

Brian Klepper, PhD, is a health care analyst and principal of Worksite Health Advisors, based in Orange Park, Florida.

Key Take-aways

- Rural employers benefit when they shop for the highest value care outside of their town if their local hospital charges monopolist rates for sub-optimal care.
- Happier and healthier employees is good for the employee and the organization's bottom-line.
- Saving on health care allowed jobs to be saved during the recession that hit the building industry especially hard.

CHAPTER 13

THE 7 HABITS OF HIGHLY EFFECTIVE BENEFITS PROFESSIONALS

"Don't mistake activity for achievement" – John Wooden

In previous chapters, I've highlighted tricks the status quo health care industry uses to redistribute profits from American companies to its coffers. Here, I will outline some basic antidotes that the most effective benefits leaders use to ensure their organizations don't needlessly overspend on health benefits.

Collectively, the approaches outlined below have enabled employers to sustainably save 20 percent or more on health benefits over the status quo.

Habit #1: Insist on Value-Based Primary Care

This is the bedrock of the highest-functioning health systems. Primary care providers own the patient relationship, are highly trusted by patients, and when properly incentivized, can be the first line of defense against downstream costs. Proper primary care is the best bulwark against inappropriate treatment pathways, including opioid overuse. Here are some of the characteristics of value-based primary care providers. They:

- Are always available in one form or another
- Welcome and immediately address complaints
- Practice shared decision making with patients
- Adequately inform patients of the risks, costs, and invasive nature of all relevant treatment options
- Refer to specialists only as necessary and only to high-value ones
- Incorporate behavioral health and physical therapy into comprehensive primary care
- Close the loop when patients are seen by specialists or are admitted to inpatient care
- Are supported by nurse practitioners and physician assistants
- Offer care in convenient locations
- Offer direct contracted care arrangements that align their economic incentives with lowering costs and improving health outcomes

Habit #2: Proactively Manage Pharmacy Benefits

Successful Rx management has been described as playing whack-a-mole. Many pharmacy benefits management (PBM) firms are well known for hidden fees, shell game pricing, and taking drug manufacturers' money to promote specific drugs. You need to stay ahead of all of these tricks.

There are four pillars to effectively managing drug costs, appropriateness, and quality:

1. Review PBM arrangements to determine the "spread" (PBM profit) and whether more favorable terms are available.
2. Make formulary changes that have a large financial impact with next to no disruption.
3. Carefully manage specialty drug purchase costs by shopping around.
4. Ensure appropriateness of prescribing to avoid overuse such as what has happened with opioids.

Habit #3: Have Specific Plans for Uncommon (But Predictable) Gargantuan Claims

You need a defined program for each common category of uncommon claims. It's not unusual for six percent of employees to account for 80 percent of total annual claim costs. They usually fall into these areas.

- **Dialysis** – With the rise of diabetes, this is inevitable. The best dialysis cost containment vendors offer multiple solutions aimed at setting the optimal price before treatment starts. They provide the most flexibility for choosing approaches that are appropriate to your specific situation.
- **Organ transplants, cancer, and complex surgery** – Sending beneficiaries to high-performance centers of excellence like Mayo Clinic and Virginia Mason Hospital & Medical Center will reduce unnecessary complications and procedures, saving enormous money despite travel costs.
- **Premature babies** – A comprehensive and closely monitored prenatal program is always worth it, especially if your employees have risk factors like advanced maternal age, diabetes, hypertension, and HIV.

Habit #4: Deploy Evidence-based Musculoskeletal (MSK) Management Programs

Given that MSK issues frequently account for 20 percent of total claim costs and that over 50 percent of procedures are not evidence-based,[124] this is a tremendous opportunity to slash costs and ill-advised overtreatment. As we saw in Chapter 6, one manufacturer increased its earnings by 1.7 percent by getting just a third of employees' MSK cases into an evidence-based management program. The impact on the company's market cap was tens of millions of dollars.

Evidence-based approaches build on clinical knowledge with modern quality management techniques and data analytics. The results, validated in many settings, demonstrate far superior health outcomes.

It's official: opioids for chronic musculoskeletal pain are a bad idea. Prescription opioid abuse is causing so many deaths by overdose that the American Centers for Disease Control and Prevention (CDC) decided it had to do something. Among their recommendations: opioids should not be considered an option for chronic musculoskeletal pain.[125]

Habit #5: Refuse to Sign Blank Checks to the Health Care Industry

Pricing failure is the most vexing problem in health care. True price transparency is the answer, e.g., bundled payments for the complete continuum of care for things like hip and knee replacements. You should demand nothing less. Virtually every area of the health care industry has high-integrity and high-quality providers that are happy to provide transparency. Find them and work with them. The Health Rosetta will help.

Habit #6: Protect Employees by Sending Them to Providers with First-rate Safety Records

In his book *Unaccountable*, Dr. Marty Makary, professor of surgery at Johns Hopkins, pointed out in devastating detail how flawed the safety culture is—and how hidden the failures are—in too many hospitals. No corporate travel department would allow an employee to fly on an airline that suppressed its safety records (even if the FAA allowed it). In the same way, it's unconscionable to blindly send an employee to a hospital with little or no information on its safety record. If the hospital suppresses that information, go elsewhere and tell your employees why.

Habit #7: Avoid Reckless Plan Document Language that Costs Millions

As mundane as ERISA plan language can sound, the most effective benefits leaders go over it with a fine-toothed comb. This is such an important topic that we've included sample document language in the Health Rosetta. You can read all about it in Chapter 26.

All your moves to implement these habits should be properly documented for two reasons. First, you want your entire team (not to mention your successor) on the same page. Second, not doing so can leave you and your company vulnerable to litigation related to health plan design and administration.

Key Take-aways

- There is no high-function health care system in the world *not* built on the foundation of great primary care. Primary care that has been devastated as badly as the United States' must be rebuilt from the ground up. Efforts to tweak the undermined primary care system have failed.
- Counter-measures must exist and be regularly updated for each high cost area such as pharmacy, musculoskeletal, and cancer. Every day, the industry develops new approaches to extract as much as possible from your organization and your employees' bottom-line.
- Smart health benefits keep people out of harm's way. For example, hospitals that suppress safety data and are more focused on building new medical complexes than patient safety should be excluded from benefits plans.

CHAPTER 14

CENTERS OF EXCELLENCE OFFER A GOLDEN OPPORTUNITY

Tom Emerick

"Don't practice until you get it right. Practice until you can't get it wrong." – Unknown

As we have seen, there is a lot of unnecessary surgery and care performed in this country. This became a particular concern for me as a benefits manager in the 1980s when I was managing BP's self-insured U.S. health plans out of its Cleveland, Ohio office. I saw employees and their family members undergoing what seemed to me to be dubious procedures. This was not the case, so far as I could see, at the Cleveland Clinic, which was used by many BP plan enrollees. So, I set up a meeting with Cleveland Clinic executives to find out why.

Basically, they explained that their ethical standards prevented them from doing surgery on patients who did not need it. Furthermore, they had an evidence-based model for diagnosing patients with great accuracy and for prescribing the safest and least invasive effective solutions.

Clearly, steering our people their way was in our employees' best interests and would lead to better outcomes for our plan members and lower health care costs for BP. As the quote above suggests, it's also critical to send individuals needing complex procedures to those with the greatest amount of experience.

What Is a Center of Excellence?

A health care solution being adopted by savvy employers across the country today is to send employees to the highest quality medical centers in the country for complex medical procedures. These centers of excellence are commonly used for cancer, neurology, cardiac care, joint replacements, and organ transplants. A center of excellence typically offers the complete continuum of care for a chronic disease or acute condition such as diabetes or breast cancer, from diagnosis to treatment to rehabilitation, at lower costs than less capable providers.

These centers are fundamentally focused on patient care more so than on research or education, although they likely do both. They practice medicine using a team-based, data-driven, and accountable model. They perform high volumes of complex surgeries with great outcomes, yet they are more likely to recommend nonsurgical treatment plans whenever appropriate.

Employers that contract directly with centers of excellence are able to offer their plan members the best care at the best price. So that's what I did. I set up what was, at that time, the largest directly contracted preferred provider network in the United States. I put the Cleveland Clinic in as the primary referral center of excellence. And, sure enough, surgery rates, almost across the board, dropped considerably.

Again, excellent diagnostics is a key to making this strategy work. Over the last 30 years, I have compiled data from various sources on patients who were sent to first-class referral centers for second opinions.

The following is a list of serious health conditions and the typical misdiagnosis rates.

- New cancer cases—20 percent
- Spine surgery—67 percent
- Orthopedic surgery—up to 30 percent
- Bypass surgery—60 percent
- Stents—50 percent in some parts of the United States.
- Solid organ transplants—40 percent

What to Look for in a Center of Excellence

Here are some of the traits that distinguish centers of excellence.

- Patients are seen by multiple specialists.
- A multidisciplinary team does the diagnosis.
- That same team prescribes the treatment plan.
- If surgery is required, it is done at the highest quality available.
- The patient experience is excellent.
- Health care is integrated, collaborative, and accountable.
- Bundled payments and global fees are the rule, rather than fee-for-service payments.

Health City in the Caymans Islands is emerging as possibly the best diagnostic and surgery center in the Western Hemisphere. A few other centers of excellence include Mayo Clinic in Minnesota, Virginia Mason in Washington, Mercy Hospital in Missouri, Intermountain Healthcare in Utah, Kaiser Permanente in California, Geisinger Health in Pennsylvania, and Baptist Health in Arkansas.

Remember that organizations are usually only a center of excellence for certain procedures and specialties, not for everything.

The High Cost of Outliers

In health benefit plans today, about six to eight percent of plan members are spending 80 percent of the plan dollars. Outliers may have wildly different medical conditions, but they have a lot in common.

- They tend to have complex health problems, usually with multiple comorbidities.
- They are often seeing three or four specialists, who rarely collaborate.
- In any given year, about 20 percent of the outlier group is completely misdiagnosed. This means that about 16 percent of plan dollars each year are being wasted on treatments for diseases the patients don't have.
- About 40 percent of outliers have treatment plans that are flat out erroneous or clearly suboptimal. Adding this to misdiagnosis means that about 32 percent of total plan dollars each year are wasted, not to mention the huge amount of medical harm to the outlier population.
- Only a handful of outlier health problems are preventable in any real sense—about seven percent, according to my colleague, Al Lewis. While the notion of workplace wellness and prevention was a noble idea, we now know that company after company is spending a huge amount of plan dollars and resources trying to do something that can't be done.

A senior executive at a Fortune 10 company wisely told me that misdiagnosis is the biggest health care error; everything that follows both harms the patient and costs you.

Those who succeed in controlling plan costs in the future will do so by focusing on outliers. One of the best solutions is using centers of excellence and taking advantage of superior referral centers to help ensure outliers are correctly diagnosed and given the optimal treatment plan.

In a typical center of excellence model, an employer pays the travel expenses for a patient and companion to travel to the center if it isn't local. If the patient needs surgery, he or she will have it at the center on the same trip. Even if the center is in another country, the quality of care more than makes up for the travel costs.

Getting Help

Admittedly, contracting directly with health systems that qualify to be centers of excellence usually takes a lot of effort, and you have to be a pretty large employer to get their attention. The good news is that "aggregators" are available today. These are specialty referral networks that can help employees of self-insured companies get prepackaged access to top-notch centers of excellence.

Some employers who have expressed an interest in working with directly contracted centers of excellence have been unsuccessful in getting support from their brokers. There is growing evidence that some benefits firms have conflicts of interest in this arena; that is, they derive a large share of their total revenue by providing consulting services that refer only to specific providers. If a broker is getting 30 percent of their total revenue in this way, they may not want to help you send your patients somewhere else.

Is your broker in this category?

Tom Emerick is a consultant on health care benefits administration, founder of Edison Health, and coauthor of Cracking Health Costs *and* An Illustrated Guide to Personal Health. *He previously led benefits programs at some of the largest employers in the world such as BP and Burger King.*

Key Take-aways

- There are extraordinary rates of misdiagnosis and overtreatment that puts patients in harm's way.
- The highest quality centers have a team-based model that allows for more accurate diagnoses and more appropriate treatment plans.
- The savings from avoidance of complications, misdiagnosis, and overtreatment more than pay for the extra cost of travel to world-class centers.

CHAPTER 15

INDEPENDENT CLAIMS ADMINISTRATORS VS. INSURANCE CARRIER OWNED CLAIMS ADMINISTRATORS – THE TRADE-OFFS

Adam V. Russo and Ron E. Peck

"The most difficult thing is to recognize that sometimes we too are blinded by our own incentives. Because we don't see how our conflicts of interest work on us." – Dan Ariely

An increasing number of employers are looking to self-insure their employee health benefits for the first time. While this is a great first step toward better benefits and lower costs, it's important to realize that not all self-insuring is the same. It can vary enormously, depending upon whether you decide to work with an insurance carrier providing administrative services only (ASO) or an independent third-party administrator (TPA).

A self-insured health plan is established when an employer sets aside some of its funds to pay for employees' medical expenses. Employees then contribute to the plan rather than pay traditional premiums. How does this differ from "insurance" as most people know it? With fully-funded "traditional" insurance, your organization pays premiums to an insurance carrier and the carrier accepts the risk, meaning the carrier pays all medical bills with its own funds. If the premiums exceed the medical expenses, the carrier "wins." If the medical expenses exceed the premiums, the carrier "loses." But for employers that can afford the risk— that have access to sufficient funds to pay the foreseeable medical expenses incurred by plan participants, as well as the occasional midsized to large dollar claim—self-insuring has been shown to be less costly overall.

A self-insured employer enjoys the following benefits:

- Plan Control — Choose what to cover and exclude, customizing the plan to be generous where your particular membership needs it, and stingy where it doesn't.
- Interest and Cash Flow — Funds are in the employer's hands until they're needed, meaning interest on those assets belongs to the employer.
- Federal Preemption and Lower Taxes — The Employee Retirement Income Security Act of 1974 states that a private, self-insured health plan is administered in accordance with its terms and federal rules. So, these plans aren't subject to conflicting state health insurance regulations or benefit mandates.
- Data — Employers can examine the claims data, study trends, allocate resources and form partnerships to address their needs.
- Risk Reduction — Reducing risk and costs directly impacts the employer and employees. Risk posed by other populations doesn't impact the plan — so employees have lower single and family premiums than those with fully funded insurance.

Overall, a self-insured plan sees net savings over a three- to five-year span, compared to a similar fully funded insurance policy.

Yet, there are risks. Among them: difficulty handling complicated claims, the threat of catastrophic claims, inability to fund claims, and new fiduciary responsibilities to members of the plan.

As mentioned, when an organization self-insures its health plan, it uses its own money plus employee contributions to pay claims for medical services. But rarely does such an organization have the resources or know-how necessary to process claims—to receive, interpret, and pay medical bills. Nor does it understand the intricacies involved in creating and managing a health plan while complying with applicable laws. Thus, an ASO or TPA is required to process and pay claims with the self-insured plan sponsor's money.

Second, while most self-insured plans have adequate resources to pay most everyday medical expenses, few have enough in hand to cover the cost of catastrophic claims resulting from care of patients with cancer, hemophilia, premature birth, etc. To address this, a self-insured plan will purchase a form of financial reinsurance or excess coverage from a stop-loss carrier. This is not health insurance in the traditional sense. The stop-loss carrier does not pay medical bills or deal directly with providers of health care. Instead, the self-insured plan—the employer—pays the medical bills. But once you have paid a certain amount (referred to as the specific deductible, attachment point, or "spec"), you can seek reimbursement from the stop-loss carrier for every dollar the plan subsequently spends beyond that "spec" deductible.

Finally, a self-insured employer acts as — or appoints — a plan administrator, who is a "fiduciary" of the plan and its members. Law dictates the fiduciary must act prudently, protect the plan and apply its terms judiciously. Failure to comply with these terms, mismanaging plan assets or doing something not in the plan's best interest could expose the plan sponsor to claims of fiduciary breach — and steep penalties. Fortunately, third-party organizations exist to step in, aid in decision-making and act as a fiduciary — indemnifying the self-insured plan administrator.

Now, let's review how a potential "self-insured" employer decides who will help them on this journey...

Note: at various times in this discussion, we will refer to the employer as the *plan sponsor* or the *client*. Employees are also called *plan members*, while members and their plan-eligible dependents are collectively called "participants."

ASO and TPA at a Glance

The traditional and simplest way to administer a self-insured plan calls for a large insurance carrier to shed its risk-bearing role but continue to serve as the employer's claims processor, substituting the employer's money for its own. This is an administrative services only or "ASO" arrangement.

ASOs prefer to pick and hire the stop-loss themselves and provide a predetermined health plan that aligns with its own stop-loss and preferred provider only (PPO) network agreements. This bundling of the plan document, stop-loss insurance, and network agreements severely limits plan customization. On the other hand, it eliminates potential gaps in coverage between these components, and makes for a relatively peaceful experience.

The transition from a fully-insured health plan to a self-insured plan is easier with an ASO, because the insurer:

- Can continue to provide the same administration expertise it provided before, including the actuarial evaluation of how much money it will cost the employer to fund its own program;
- Can provide other professional services such as accounting, legal advice, expert medical opinions, and regulatory compliance;
- Is usually familiar with the medical providers known to the employees and with employees' health risks, both important to handling claims; and, as mentioned…
- Ensures the plan, stop-loss, and network all abide by the same terms.

The downside is that the employer can't take as much of an active role in cost management or provider relations. Nor can it easily negotiate a direct contract with a hospital or "carve out" a particular type of claim. In return for one-stop shopping, you generally do what the ASO dictates, limiting your flexibility to significantly reduce spending.

With a TPA, on the other hand, you call the shots and get more transparency and flexibility for what is generally a lower cost. The TPA does what you dictate.

As benefit plans have become more sophisticated and self-insuring more popular, we've seen a nationwide proliferation of increasingly professional TPAs. These independent administrators offer a broad range of services. At one end is the simple administration of benefit payments. At the other is a "turn-key" contract that includes a stop-loss provision like an ASO but is still more flexible and affordable.

Due to consolidation, there are fewer small "boutique" TPAs these days, but even the larger TPAs dominating the market still maintain more of a customized approach than an ASO. They are more flexible, more likely to be local, and offer employers the opportunity to access claims data. They also let you pick and choose vendors and providers to meet your specific usage needs. Thanks to their highly specialized products and lower overhead, TPAs have developed pricing strategies that make them cost-effective. A TPA can afford medical expertise and achieve group purchasing discounts that are significantly more advantageous than those available to a single employer. More employers are finding that it's worth risking potential gaps in coverage with a TPA, in exchange for being able to shop around and field offers from various stop-loss carriers.

Also, ASOs are generally proprietary regarding claims data. If you as the employer want to know if your smoking cessation program has yielded an ROI, it can be hard to get the data needed to see the changes. If you want to examine your costs for diabetes treatment before deciding on a program for Type 2 diabetics, it can be hard to get data. With a TPA, you have complete access to the data, allowing you to design your plan accordingly. Increasingly, employers believe it's unconscionable to not have visibility into what is likely their organization's biggest expenditure after payroll.

Here's another difference. Many self-insured plans place great emphasis on their preferred provider organization (PPO). (See Chapter 8 PPO for more on PPOs and how they are responsible for keeping health costs so high.) This is a prearranged network of pro-viders that agree to treat plan members for a discounted rate and to accept that amount as payment in full. The biggest networks are owned and managed by large insurance carriers, but nevertheless provide access to their own insurance programs and ASO plans. On the other hand, even when TPAs "rent" networks from large carriers, the carriers do not provide their deepest discounts to any-one outside their own organization.

Thus, some TPAs are forgoing the national network approach, instead focusing on direct contracting with individual providers for even better rates and/or forming high quality networks of select providers for rates that rival or beat the best national PPOs. The downside, of course, is that if plan members go outside the high-quality network for treatment, they can be billed out of pocket for the balance after the plan pays the maximum amount allowable according to the contract—something that doesn't hap-pen if the plan and provider are part of a national PPO.

With a TPA, there is a true unbundling of services. For some employers, the fact that a TPA requires the employer to see and select the moving parts is exciting. It allows a hands-on employer to more actively contain costs and pick what they feel is best for their employees. For others, it is frightening and overwhelming. For those employers, an ASO that makes the decisions for them is likely the way to go—if they're willing to pay the premium.

ASO Benefits

There are a lot of parts to administering a benefits plan and an ASO will take care of all of them;

- Accounting and recordkeeping
- Plan design
- Actuarial analysis
- Underwriting
- Securing stop-loss coverage
- Investment advice

- Enrollment
- Utilization review
- Medical record audits
- Plan booklet preparation
- COBRA administration
- Plan communication
- Reporting and disclosure
- Contribution determination
- Claims administration
- Statistical analysis
- Subrogation
- Claim appeals
- Record retention

The ASO will also decide whether, when, and how much to pay for claims.

Of late, insurance carriers, including their ASO arms, have improved their service capabilities, making them more transparent. In some cases, it is possible for a self-insured employer to log onto an ASO's technology platform and instantly receive claims status reports—for an extra cost, mind you.

As self-insuring has become more important in the market, some insurance carriers also have implemented programs to make their products easier to use. This revolution in customer service includes onsite processing personnel, 800 numbers, artificial intelligence systems, image processing, and other advanced technology designed to generate one-call responses to member inquiries.

Self-insuring with an ASO is truly a turn-key solution. You and your employees enjoy a seamless transition from fully-insured traditional insurance. There are no gaps between the plan's coverage and stop-loss coverage. Yet there is a cost for this all-in-one approach. In addition to administrative fees that admittedly range but almost always exceed the fees charged by TPAs (sometimes doubling them), your rights to examine data and customize your plan, as well as pick and choose stop-loss carriers and vendors, is limited, and stop-loss insurance premiums are usually greater. This arrangement, together with bundled pharmacy services, significantly limits your ability to proactively and significantly reduce your total spending.

TPA Benefits

Different types of TPAs have different strengths. On large accounts, for example, the large nationwide TPAs can compete favorably with large insurers' ASO-driven products. Smaller, local TPAs can generally respond more quickly to plan changes than their larger counterparts.

Interacting and working with a TPA on a local level can bring a high degree of control to the administrative process. A TPA located in the same community as an employer has the advantages of knowing the market, employees, providers, and general economic conditions. This familiarity can lead to administrative and benefits efficiencies. If the TPA is part of a local managed care organization, serving other employers, it has a stronger negotiating position.

A thorough knowledge and understanding of the labor market and the benefits available locally for various employee classifications will also help in planning benefits. This means the TPA will be competitive and likely to achieve the goals of the employers' overall benefit strategy.

Two other advantages that TPAs have over ASOs are negotiating "in network" claims and changing terms in the summary plan description (SPD). Because many ASOs are affiliated with the PPO network they use (often sharing a parent company or other affiliation), they are typically expected to process all in-network claims quickly—without examining them. While quick and painless claims payments certainly limit conflicts with providers and insured individuals, they also make it more likely that excessive charges, duplicate and fraudulent claims, and other billing errors will be missed.

Recently, a TPA processing claims for its self-insured plan client performed an audit on in-network claims (something an

ASO might not be allowed to do) and discovered a $3.6 million claim *after* the network discount. The claim featured many coding and other mistakes, but once these were addressed, the final payment was a much more manageable $1.6 million!

Whether because the claims processing system is keyed to work with a particular benefit plan template, or because applicable network and stop-loss policies are written in concert with the plan document, many ASO-managed plans are stuck with a predetermined SPD document. For many self-insured employers, this is a great comfort. For others, the lack of discretionary authority is troublesome. In one case, an employer working with an ASO was strongly opposed to paying for claims arising from all illegal acts. The plan document excluded only claims arising from felonies. When the employer asked to expand the scope to all illegal acts, he was told that such a change would disrupt coordination with the claims system, stop-loss, and network contracts.

As cost containment and managed care become increasingly important, the balance is tipping toward the TPAalternative.

Another Consideration: Are You Hiring an Independent Advocate?

Whether ASO or TPA, some claims processors are partly owned by large insurance carriers, health systems, network administrators, and other entities. This means that when you want to dispute something with one of those entities, their claims processor may need to bow out due to conflict of interest. In one instance, a small employer's plan members were being asked by a local hospital to pay a portion of their bill *upfront* because the plan didn't use a recognized provider network. The hospital was not hassling members of other, much larger area employer plans administered by the same TPA and likewise not using a network. The TPA confronted the hospital on the plan's behalf, leveraging the weight of all of its clients to force the hospital to explain the issues and devise a better solution. Had the TPA been beholden to the hospital, this wouldn't have happened.

In another instance, the employer sponsoring a self-insured plan was questioning a hospital's billing practices. When it refused to pay the full billed charges, the hospital returned the plan's partial payment, threatening to "balance bill" the individual directly for 100 percent of the billed charges.

Had the plan been working with a TPA or ASO that was affiliated with the hospital, it almost certainly would have pushed the employer to reissue payment in accordance with the network terms. But because the TPA was entirely independent, it agreed to issue the plan's maximum allowable payment directly to the individual. In addition, it hired an advocate to represent the individual in negotiating with the hospital. By taking these steps, the individual, employer, and TPA were able to get the provider to abandon a two percent discount in favor of a 35 percent discount, saving almost $30,000.

A Closer Look at Fiduciary Responsibility

One benefit inherent in an ASO approach relates to fiduciary duties. A self-insured employer, unlike an employer purchasing a fully-insured health plan, is deemed to be a fiduciary of the plan members. This means he or she is legally bound to act prudently and only in their interest. Actions that are deemed to be in error, arbitrary, or capricious can expose employers to treble damages, that is, penalties are sometimes equal to three times the damage caused. For many employers, who have never taken on a fiduciary role, this is intimidating and not welcome. Often, an ASO is willing to take on that role with you.

With TPAs, things are less straightforward. A TPA is a contract service provider, not a plan administrator. The administrator role is reserved for the employer or trustee-appointed fiduciary. However, TPAs increasingly are taking on plan administrator functions—and with them, apparently, increased liability.

For example, TPAs are promoting programs such as Multiple Employer Welfare Arrangements or "MEWAs," which are statutorily regulated plans comprised of multiple smaller employers banding together, moving into marketing, stop-loss procurement, and consulting services. In response, TPAs are coming under scrutiny for their handling of plan funds and invested assets. Courts already have found some traditional claims administration functions to be of a fiduciary nature—particularly regarding handling and management of plan assets—and have held TPAs accountable as functional fiduciaries under the higher standards of conduct. Some states have attempted to regulate TPA services as a form of insurance business. However, a number of courts have held that state regulation of TPAs—and of self-insured plans—is preempted by ERISA (the Employee Retirement Income Security Act of 1974).

Even if you hand over fiduciary duties to a TPA or ASO, ERISA says you may remain liable for its breach of its duties *if,* say, there are no procedures in the plan to delegate those duties. But if there are procedures and you follow them, you will be held responsible for the TPA's misconduct *only if you failed to exercise prudence in selecting the TPA or monitoring their performance.*

Naturally, you will want to consult an attorney in this matter.

Empowered Plans

One often overlooked, but certainly underappreciated aspect of self-insuring is the sense of ownership the employer and employees should have over their program. Indeed, when we pay "premiums" to a carrier, and shift the risk inherent in claims payment onto that carrier, we don't really think twice about how much this MRI or that vaccine costs. In fact, like someone at the all-you-can-eat buffet who skips past the veggies and eats nothing but lobster tail, we want to get all we can get for our money. Our premiums are already set in stone, so let's stick it to the carrier by spending as much as possible on our care. With a self-insured plan, however, a dollar saved is a dollar earned by the employer and employees.

Not every self-insured employer truly takes this to heart, however, and fails to educate their staff regarding how their actions and inaction can impact how much they all spend on care. An empowered plan, however, will take steps to do just that. Consider a plan that – on its own – identifies the hospitals in its area, and (by examining the data) determines which generally charge more than the others to deliver a baby. Next, they take the reasonably priced facilities and research the quality outcomes published annually, to identify which are the safest as well as best priced.

With those two metrics in hand, this empowered plan has identified "centers of excellence," and notifies its staff that if a woman on the plan chooses to deliver their baby at one of these select facilities, the employer will pay for the baby's diapers and wipes for a year. That is a win-win scenario for both the participant and the plan.

Looking back on the issues discussed, we see how the use of an ASO versus a TPA can impact a plan's ability to achieve "empowered" status. The employer had to examine the data (recall we discussed how an ASO may be more protective of the data than a TPA), and the employer may potentially be incentivizing staff to visit one "in-network" provider over another... something the PPO (and thus the ASO carrier) may not be thrilled with.

This is just one example of how a hands-on self-insured plan can take cost containment to the next level, and how the decision of whom to work with, as it relates to plan administration, will impact those efforts.

Ready to Get Started?
A Checklist for Decision Makers

Here are some reasons you might decide to self-insure.

1. **Plan control.** You choose what to cover and exclude. With a TPA, you are able to directly control costs by designing and implementing care strategies that are informed by your culture, employee behaviors, and local health and provider resources.
2. **Interest and cash flow.** Funds are in your hands until they're needed.
3. **Federal preemption and lower taxes.** ERISA states that a private, self-insured health plan isn't subject to conflicting state health insurance regulations.
4. **Data access.** You can, if you have a TPA, examine claims data, study trends, allocate resources, and form partnerships to address your company's unique needs.
5. **Risk reduction.** Reducing risk and costs directly impacts you and your employees, plus you're unaffected by other populations.

On the other hand, you and your employees may be used to a fully-insured traditional insurance policy, with all that implies: "in-network" access to providers, often nationwide; knowing those providers will accept whatever the plan dictates in terms of charges; and predetermined decisions about what is covered and what is not, and how a complicated claim should be handled.

How important are these things to you?

Take some time to consider the following before making your decision to self-insure and picking either a TPA or an ASO.

- Do you want to make the effort to compare your plan document, which you helped draft, to a stop-loss carrier's policy to be sure you won't be stuck paying certain types of claims the carrier doesn't cover? Or, would you rather some-one else handle drafting the plan and picking stop-loss?

- Do you care whether you have a nationwide network, or do you prefer local narrow networks and direct contracts, which might save you more money but expose your employees to the possibility of balance billing?
- Do you care who services your plan—who's watching the claims and who's making sure your plan is being reimbursed when someone else is supposed to pay?
- Do you care whether you're paying for services and programs your employees don't actually need or use? Are you concerned that your population has needs not being adequately addressed?
- Do you want to implement the most innovative, evidence-based practices to improve employee health and reduce waste and costs?

If you place more importance on large network discounts (albeit off of undisclosed and inflated prices and over which there are no controls), and avoiding decision making (and liability for those decisions), then you are an ideal candidate to self-insure with an ASO.

If you are willing to risk potential gaps in coverage between your plan and your stop-loss and assume liability for decision making as a fiduciary, in exchange for controlling which providers your employees have access to, what your plan covers, and which programs, vendors, and carriers you work with, then you are a prime candidate for self-insuring with a TPA.

Ron E. Peck, Esq. is senior vice president and general counsel and Adam Russo, Esq. is the cofounder and chief executive officer of The Phia Group, an organization dedicated to empowering health plans' ability to maximize benefits while minimizing costs.

What to look for in a TPA

Is the TPA able to deliver value? This can be in the following forms.

- Value-based contracting
- Integration with local primary care practices
- Chronic care management and reporting
- Cost and quality transparency
- Seamless integration and promotion of third-party solutions like telehealth or second opinions
- Flexibility in customer communication (phone only between 8am and 5pm? Or text, email, chat anytime?)

Will the TPA be able to smoothly accommodate you as a new client? One clue is the size of your company relative to the TPA's other clients.

What is the TPA's performance track record on things like turn-around time for claims processing (seven to 10 business days is average) and accuracy (look for a percentage in the upper 90s)? Reputation in the stop-loss market is a good indicator.

What do their turnover rate, past performance evaluations, reference checks, feedback from dissatisfied clients, and pending litigation tell you about the performance of individual staff who will administer your program?

Is the TPA's technology sophisticated enough to account for and appropriately allocate the cost of benefits, provide a superior customer experience, and evaluate both the cost of the various benefits being offered and the efficiencies of providers? (In many cases, the answer is no.)

Does the TPA have a strong relationship with a stop-loss carrier that might help sway excess coverage reimbursements in your favor?

Is the TPA able to meet the competing demands of federal privacy rules and Department of Labor claims procedures rules that accelerate the decision-making process? Can it meet HIPAA's standardization requirements for electronic codes and formats?

Is the TPA prepared in terms of technological capabilities and capital resources to operate in the ever-more demanding compliance environment?

Key Take-aways

- Carrier-control claims administration, for a self-insured employer, operate nearly identically to a traditional insurance program. That is an advantage and disadvantage.
- Carrier-provided claims administration severely impair your ability to maintain cost control and prevent employees from going to provider organizations with poor value and safety records.
- Independently administered benefits plans are more work. However, they offer a limitless ability to ensure that plan beneficiaries receive the greatest value and patient safety. Employers spending 20 percent less (or ever deeper savings) per capita, while providing superior benefits, all use independent administrators.

CHAPTER 16

THE FUTURE OF HEALTH WILL BE LOCAL, OPEN, AND INDEPENDENT

"All of us are smarter than any of us." – Douglas Merrill

It should come as no surprise that the most successful solutions to society's most challenging problems do not now and will not in the future arrive with the cavalry from Washington, D.C. After all, the great societal challenges that America has been tackling over the last several decades—civil rights, energy independence, climate change, better food—all have been fueled from the bottom-up.

This is certainly true when it comes to health care: an industry that spends more on lobbying than oil and gas, defense, and financial services *combined* is going to have its way with Congress. [126] I've taken to calling most D.C. politicos "preservatives" rather than progressives or conservatives, as they get paid to preserve the status quo. The fact remains that over the last couple decades neither Democrats nor Republicans have accomplished much to address the two biggest failings of the U.S. health care system—pricing failure and overtreatment.

Health care is particularly suited to a bottom-up approach because it begins at home. The fundamental value creation in health care is the relationship between an individual and his or her care team. The more intermediaries and bureaucrats that get inserted into that relationship, the greater the chance for value to be extracted rather than added.

Venture capitalist Chris Brookfield has close to 20 years' experience in emerging markets investing and entrepreneurship in the telecom sector. In 2004, he left mainstream venture capital to focus on investments with broader and more beneficial human impact. He and his team played an instrumental role in lifting tens of millions out of poverty through microfinance, small business loans, rural hospital development, and slum improvement finance in India. He is now applying his systems change model to remaking the U.S. food system through a new financial instrument he's calling full circle capital. (See Appendix B for the full text of Brookfield's white paper, "A Practical Handbook for Systems Change.")

Tired political labels get swept aside when people come together to solve their issues. Brookfield's work in food has revealed a natural collaboration between farmers and those in the local food movement, even though farmers tend to be more politically conservative and local food people tend to be more politically progressive. We find the same thing in health care, where free market-oriented, conservative physicians are pursuing the same objectives and using similar tactics as progressive union leaders.

Models that deliver systemic change, says Brookfield, have three big themes in common: They're local, open, and independent. In this chapter, I'm going to show how health care can capitalize on these same themes, using excerpts from Brookfield's paper (shown in italics).

Local

By focusing on local, a number of intrinsic advantages are often overlooked. First, by decreasing scale, solutions can appear to problems that seem too complicated to solve at the global scale. For instance, re-engineering the food system or decreasing poverty really are intractable when viewed at the global scale. Even the basic atoms of these systems—people—are invisible. By dialing into local, new features and relationships emerge.

In their new book, *The New Localism*, urban experts Bruce Katz and Jeremy Nowak describe a diversity of needs at the local level. They compare cities such as Detroit, which may need to demolish blighted housing to boost value, to hot market cities such as Boston, which may need to build and preserve more housing to meet demand. State and federal legislatures tend to enact one-size-fits-all solutions and, often for political reasons, prefer spreading public resources evenly, despite widely varying needs. New localism allows communities to focus on the challenges they actually have rather than on the national issue "du jour".

Localism realigns entrenched politics. It's striking how new alliances are formed at the local level that are impossible at the national level, where conservatives see new federalism, independence, entrepreneurism, and local business, and progressives see community building, health, nutrition, education, and nurturing. In health care, individuals receive care from local clinicians, yet less than 25 cents of every dollar spent goes to these locally-based, value-creating clinicians. Between 50 and 75 cents of every dollar goes to health systems and health plans that are usually headquartered elsewhere. This is at the heart of how the "sick care" industry has extracted resources that would otherwise go to social determinants of health that are fundamentally local (e.g., schools and social services). The table below shows where the health care dollar goes.

~$0.45	Fraud	Extractive or no value
	Misdiagnosis & overtreatment	
	(High cost, massive overtreatment: spinal & stent procedures; high misdiagnosis areas: oncology, musculoskeletal, etc., ranging from 25% to 67%)	
	Abusive & arbitrarily high prices	
	(Massive pricing failure: prices for similar quality often vary 2-10x)	
~$0.30	Insurer or health system administration & overhead	Often extractive
~$0.25	Paying high-value care providers	Generally not extractive

Note: *These are very high-level approximations for illustrative purposes. They're based on multiple, widely recognized sources and generally accepted data, including PwC's "The price of excess - identifying waste in health care spending" and Institute of Medicine's*[127] *estimate of waste at 30-50 percent of spending. Other data points are outlined elsewhere in the book, including rates of misdiagnosis and pricing failure.*

One of the key architects of the ACA, Bob Kocher, MD, echoes these lessons learned in a *Wall Street Journal* op-ed[128] entitled "How I Was Wrong About Obamacare," in which he outlines the importance of independent, locally controlled medical practices.

"Personal relationships of the kind found in smaller practices are the key to the practice of medicine. Small, independent practices know their patients better than any large health system ever can… [They] are able to change their care models in weeks and rapidly learn how to use data to drive savings and quality… [I]t does not take [them] years to root out waste, rewire referrals to providers who charge less but deliver more, and redesign schedules so patients can see their doctors more often to avert emergency-room visits and readmissions.

"I believed then that the consolidation of doctors into larger physician groups was inevitable and desirable under the ACA. What I know now, though, is that having every provider in health care 'owned' by a single organization is more likely to be a barrier to better care."

Open

Openness is an advantage, largely because information networks have coalesced over the past 15 years and have exponentially increased the flow of information to local communities. There is no way to transmit proprietary ideas at anywhere near the speed and coverage that open sourced ideas move.

Openness is proving itself in an array of settings. The beer market is mature and has been dominated in the U.S. by a couple behemoths, yet craft brewers recently have grabbed over 20 percent[129] of beer spending. How? Craft brewers are radically open with each other regarding how to succeed, recognizing that their real competition is the mega brewers, not each other.

One of the failings of the wildly underperforming status quo health care system is how poorly insights and breakthroughs get disseminated. Research shows that it takes 17 years[130] for effective breakthroughs to become mainstream. This is why a central tenet of the Health Rosetta is to create an open, Wikipedia-like "hive mind" that makes it much easier to understand and deploy approaches that sustainably outperform traditional approaches to Quadruple Aim objectives.

Near the conclusion of a great new book, *Our Towns*, James Fallows echoed the theme of taking what's already working and sharing it much more broadly. He quotes Philip Zelikow, a professor at the University of Virginia who said to Fallows: "In scores of ways, Americans are figuring out how to take advantage of the opportunities of this era, often through bypassing or ignoring the dismal national conversation. There are a lot of more positive narratives out there – but they're lonely, and disconnected. It would make a difference to join them together, as a chorus that has a melody."

Katz and Nowak describe a new circuitry of civic innovation, in which innovative practices are adapted from one city to another – cities in radically different circumstances that are simultaneously trying to solve similar challenges. The adaptation of solutions is accelerated by new city-related associations that share innovation, industry-specific organizations such as the Health Rosetta, or major foundations such as the Rockefeller Foundation.

Independent

As with scale, we are hybridizing our approach to system design [of next-generation wheat mills] to incorporate the best of both local and conglomerated infrastructure. By integrating business models with existing social movements, we achieve network connectivity beyond the local watershed, allowing the sharing of resources, information and values. By allowing each of these businesses to function autonomously within this fabric and grow to their fullest individual potentials, an individual mill can utilize the control and hierarchical scalability typified by corporation... [A]t the same time, the fabric as a whole achieves quick responses, flexibility, and adaptability – responses which are inhibited by corporate concentration.

The first broad application of the local, open, and independent model is the vanguard benefits advisors who are the torchbearers of the next health era. Perhaps no job is more underestimated in all of health care in terms of its potential to help (or hurt) the working and middle class of America. Our experience has been that the vast majority of employers defer most of their health benefit decision-making to their benefits broker / consultant. As outlined elsewhere in the book, this is often to the detriment of employers and their stakeholders, whether they be employees, shareholders, taxpayers, or otherwise.

The Health Rosetta certified benefits advisors are building the next generation health economy by replicating what is proving successful in a wide array of settings: public and private employers, rural and urban settings, large and small employers. Again, *replication* is the key word. Given that the primary value creation in health care is fundamentally a local endeavor tuned to local dynamics, we believe replication is the way change will happen. This is a fundamental contrast to massive top-down, large-scale programs. Replication varies from application to application;

scalability seeks to apply the same things everywhere. This distinction is a subtle but absolutely critical success factor.

Post Political

One indicator that a movement is ready for development in the commercial sphere is indicated when the movement ceases to be perceived as political within the relevant communities. While movements remain politicized, there is insufficient agreement; when the community itself is split in its support, this method of commercial development is doomed at the outset. On the other hand, it was obvious in the case of both microcredit and local food, that virtually everyone in the local communities agreed with the underlying premise. When the commercial values aligned community business models were tested, they were able to attract nearly unanimous support.

As Katz and Nowak point out, new localism is also nonpartisan—and powerful.

"The regular engagement of business, civic, and academic leaders elevates pragmatic thinking and commonsense discourse and crowds out the inflammatory rhetoric associated with partisanship and ideology. New localism is intensely focused on maximizing value for long-term prosperity rather than short-term private profit or political gain. Cities main message to the federal government today is 'first, do no harm.'

"Millions of decisions are made by subnational leaders and ordinary citizens, and these decisions build communities, drive economies, educate children, catalyze innovation, and change lives. New localism is both representative of and restorative of the democratic ideals and principles on which the republic was founded in which sustain Americans in good and bad times."

Perhaps it is time to dust off the public referenda process to garner support for transformative investments in the future. A great example of this is how the Austin electorate voted to tax itself during an economic downturn in order to fund the Dell

Medical School. Central to the mission of the new medical school is serving as the community health care provider. Even in the short time since they opened, they've tackled issues that had been poorly addressed. For example, the working poor in Austin had an 18-month wait to be seen for orthopedic issues. Today, it's down to about a week, thanks to on-the-ground problem-solving versus simply pouring more resources into a clearly flawed approach.

The way we structured health insurance was the original sin that led to the medical-industrial complex.

In *An American Sickness*, Elisabeth Rosenthal outlined how the way we structured health insurance was in some ways the original sin that catalyzed the evolution of today's medical-industrial complex. This doesn't mean health insurance is a bad thing. It means health insurance as we have known it is a bad thing. We need to re-do health insurance to support the health care system we want, not the one we've got. Brookfield believes that huge risk pools are the heart of the problem.

When local networks are scaled up, you add hierarchy, says Brookfield, and this creates opportunity for theft and redirection. Brookfield's genius has been understanding how social missions can be nested within free markets and how local control is a path to broad, positive change. This has been applied to microcredit, rural hospital development, and more. He has a proven track record of transpartisan approaches to tackling extremely difficult problems such as systemic poverty, lack of access to health care, and our food production system that has harmed local economies while producing sub-par food. The following is Brookfield's reaction to Rosenthal's comment:

All group risk pools—health insurance, life insurance, credit insurance, disaster/property insurance—have a long social history. They all evolved out of village/community mutual aid groupings. So, for instance, along with microcredit (which has analogs that go back thousands of years) there were all kinds of group risk insurance. The community would pay if one member had an unanticipated tragedy.

These systems work very well at the community level. They are efficient and well supervised (by their own participants); a semi-autonomous network operating at the local level for insurance services. In this kind of network—some call it a fabric—there is much mutual overlap. Walls are thin, and gossip travels fast. This kind of signaling among community participants is really very effective at reigning in abuses of systems connecting throughout the community. Also, because links are very short, there is not much bureaucracy, lag times, or translation errors. Close neighbors equals gossip and thin walls, which drives effective emergence of community governance. If one abuses the system of "insurance" everyone would know quickly and you would be censured. This is the essence of Elinor Ostrom's insight that won her the Nobel Prize for economics. These systems go completely haywire when "scaled up."

When this kind of local network is "scaled up" you add hierarchy (bureaucracy). This makes this kind of ad hoc governance very difficult as links are not close and additional layers create opportunity for theft and redirection.

Taken as a whole, I think it is a mistake to think of any kind of insurance as being made for the beneficiary. In nearly all cases—even the village case—the system of insurance benefits the relatives and neighbors or more distant relations of the beneficiary. In the primary case—where there is no systemic insurance—people still get help to survive their catastrophic risks. The only question is how those risks are borne and how many people carry the burden.

Persuading individuals to buy insurance is kind of backwards. I saw this in India all the time. Individuals do not value their own risks— their relatives and neighbors do. We could not get individuals to buy insurance. We made buying life insurance compulsory to receiving a much bigger benefit—personal loans. Then we quickly sold 10 million policies. And this alleviated a huge burden for our lending institutions collecting on loans from families of the deceased or their estates. The value of this insurance accrued to the lenders, first; and only secondarily to their surviving family members.

It would be good for American policy makers to be reminded that insurance is not an attractive sale to an individual b) the beneficiaries of insurance, fundamentally, are the family, community members and invested financial institutions not the insured.

Most modern insurance vastly scales up the number of people who bear the burden and, in the process, adds enormous cost while losing effective oversight.

What is the smallest actuarially valid risk pool? Several actuaries and an economist have shown me that pools over 1,000 people are redundant and may actually reduce resilience as the ballooning overheads are costlier than the marginal benefit from wider risk sharing. So why do pools end up huge, in the hundreds of thousands or more? More power and money to the administrators, plus hugely expanded cost of end of life intervention that adds a big nut for a smaller pool. Insurance administration grows scale and cost, which drives additional costs from providers...and on we turn.

For nearly all people nearly all of the time, says Brookfield, we would be better off with community risk pools, self-governed, for nearly all of our risks, using traditional pools only as reinsurance.

It would be great to create neighborhood risk pools as an alternative and use traditional pools only as reinsurance sitting behind the neighborhood pools.

The primary issue of outlier claims is easily addressed. Over 100 million Americans are in self-insured plans. All but the largest have stop-loss policies for outlier claims. This allows companies as small as 20 people to self-insure without risk of financial ruin if they have an unfortunate medical incident.

'Buy Local' Programs Will Reinvigorate Communities

Increasingly, communities realize the value of "buy local" programs that increase community resilience and economic opportunity. Today, the vast majority of communities send a large amount of money to out-of-town bureaucracies to pay for services that are mostly delivered locally. It's quite odd if you pause and think about it. In contrast, the Rosen Hotels case study is a microcosm of how a community can be literally transformed (crime down, high school graduations up, etc.) by reinvesting money that would have otherwise been squandered on giant out-of-town bureaucracies. Likewise, Pittsburgh has shown how a local insurance pool can ensure education budgets no longer get eviscerated by a wasteful health care system.

Even in countries perceived to have centralized health care systems, ownership and administration is pushed down to much more local levels. Communities like Jönköping, Sweden[131] have been internationally recognized[132] for how they innovate and reallocate monies to fit the needs of community members. Jönköping leaders are aware that clinical health care drives less than 20 percent of health outcomes, so balancing that spending with investments in clean air and water, better schools, job training, and other opportunity creation maximizes community well-being.

In many ways, we already have this today in a variety of communities, from employers (self-insured and captive) to unions to health sharing ministries. My partner, Sean Schantzen, tells me all the time about ways organizations hedge their bets against risks of all kinds, many of which are highly complex and unpredictable. For example, the wide range of reinsurance products, commodities options, currency hedging, etc. are all forms of insurance that enable organizations to tailor their protection to their comfort level with risk.

We know that our current approach to health insurance isn't well-received. Customer satisfaction with status quo health insurance is lower than virtually any other sector of the economy. The beauty of the approach Brookfield articulates is the blend of local control and accountability with the scale advantage from appropriate use of technology and modern business tools. Without local accountability, distant bureaucracies are vulnerable to abuse. Consequently, a cascade of stifling bureaucracy gets layered on to the point we've reached today. None of us want physicians spending two hours on bureaucracy for every hour of patient time, least of all physicians. The burden becomes an alphabet soup that crushes our nurses and doctors—MACRA, MIP, MU, PCMH, HCAHPS and more. Whether in the United States or abroad, I've observed that the closer a health care delivery organization is to where patients live, work, play, and pray, the better it performs and the less need there is for stifling bureaucracy. Clinicians have a direct affinity with and accountability to their patients.

People sometimes conflate re-localizing health care and health insurance with past clumsy efforts to pool risk, many of which haven't worked.[133]

They didn't work for the following reasons:

- They brought organizations together that had no connection or local accountability and were driven by distant state bureaucracies.
- They were predicated on buying from out-of-area intermediaries, insurance or provider companies versus locally-controlled provider organizations. With that came all the baggage outlined in other parts of this book, such as PPO networks that once made sense but have become value-extractors from local families and economies. Case studies throughout this book of unions, employers, and municipalities demonstrate how they are more effective than insurance companies at slashing health costs by managing things at an appropriate scale. Why? They have aligned interests absent from most intermediary arrangements in health care.
- They used the same old health payment approaches that have proven to deliver mediocre health outcomes, eat up extraordinary sums of money, and make clinicians' lives miserable. Hardly a recipe for success. When social missions are nested within free markets and local control, there is a path to broad, positive change that is embraced by people who put their humanity before tired political labels.

Key Take-aways

- By decreasing scale to a local level, solutions can appear to problems that seem too complicated to solve at the global scale.

- Roughly half of every dollar spent on health care adds no value; much of it is extracted out of local economies to out-of-town health plans, health systems, and investors, even though health care is fundamentally local. The value-creating nurses and doctors receive well under $0.25 of every dollar.
- There is no way to transmit proprietary ideas at anywhere near the speed and coverage that open sourced ideas move. The arc of health bends toward openness.
- Transforming health care requires re-doing health insurance to support the health care system we want, not the one we've got. This doesn't mean health insurance is a bad thing. It means health insurance as we have known it has created a multitude of perverse incentives that harm both patients and clinicians.
- Combining the best of local autonomy with the benefits of modern financial and technology infrastructure can be achieved in post political movements.

CHAPTER 17

HEALTH 3.0 VISION AND IMPLICATIONS FOR PROVIDERS & GOVERNMENT

"Healthy citizens are the greatest asset any country can have." — *Winston S. Churchill*

As health benefits get a major overhaul in the employer arena, and policymakers determine where publicly paid health care programs will go, we believe it's imperative to take a fresh look at how we've organized our health care system. One area of near-universal agreement is that we should expect far more from our health care system, given the smarts, money, and passion poured into it. Simply shifting who pays for care does little to address the underlying dysfunction of what we pay for and how we pay.

A group of forward-looking individuals have developed a vision for the future of health care. Health 3.0 is a common framework to guide the work of everyone from clinical leaders to benefits professionals to technologists to policymakers. Each should ask whether their strategies, technologies, and policies accelerate or hinder the journey to Health 3.0.

How is Health 3.0 different than Health Rosetta? If Health 3.0 is the North Star—where we want to be—Health Rosetta is the roadmap plus travel tips on how to get there.

Health 3.0 Encompasses Four Key Dimensions:

1. Health services (i.e., care delivery and self-care)

What is the optimal way to organize health services, so they build on the strengths of each piece of the health puzzle, rather than operating as an unmatched set of pieces as they do today? Innovative new care delivery models create a bright future that some are already experiencing, in which every member of the care team is operating at the top of his or her license and is highly satisfied with his or her role—a stark contrast to Health Care 2.0, where only 27 percent of a doctor's day is spent on clinical face-time with patients.[134]

2. Health care purchasing

Health Rosetta and Health 3.0 provide a high-level blueprint for how to purchase health and wellness services wisely. Underlying virtually every dysfunction in health care are perverse economic incentives. Remember, various industry players are acting perfectly rationally when they do things that are counterproductive to a system that delivers value to every party. We've seen how a workforce can achieve what one health care innovator has described as "twice the health care at half the cost and ten times the delight."

3. Enabling technology

Contrary to common thinking that technology alone can be a positive force for change, technology only turbocharges a highly functional organizational process when the proper organization structure, economic incentives, and processes are in place. Unfortunately, today's health care breaks the first rules I learned as a new consultant fresh out of school—don't automate a broken process and don't throw technology on top of it.

4. Enabling government

At the local, state, and federal level, government can play a tremendously beneficial (or detrimental) role in ensuring health care reaches its full potential. There are four main ways that government entities contribute:

1. As an enabler of health (e.g., public health and social determinants of health)
2. As a benefits purchaser, since government entities are large employers who can accelerate acceptance of new, higher-performing Health 3.0 care models
3. As a payer of taxpayer-funded health plans
4. As a lawmaking or regulating entity

The second item, in particular, is frequently overlooked as a powerful tool for testing and refinement of new models of care payment and delivery.

Health 3.0 Builds on Assets, Corrects Failings of Health 1.0 and 2.0

I'll let Dr. Zubin Damania (aka ZDoggMD), the founder of Health 3.0, make the comparison.[135]

Behind us lies a long-lost, nostalgia-tinged world of unfettered physician autonomy, sacred doctor-patient relationships, and a laser-like focus on the art and humanity of medicine. This was the world of my father, an immigrant and primary care physician in rural California. The world of Health care 1.0. While many still pine for these 'good old days' of medicine, we shouldn't forget that those days weren't really all that good. With unfettered autonomy came high costs and spotty quality. Evidence-based medicine didn't exist; it was consensus and intuition. Volume-based fee-for-service payments incentivized doing things to people, instead of for people. And although the relationship was sacred, the doctor often played the role of captain of the ship, with the rest of the health care team and the patients subordinate.

So, in response to these shortcomings we now have Health Care 2.0—the era of Big Medicine. Large corporate groups buying practices and hospitals, managed care and Obamacare, randomized controlled trials and evidence-based guidelines, EMRs, PQRS, HCAHPS, MACRA, Press Ganey, Lean, and Six Sigma. It is the era of Medicine as Machine...of Medicine as Assembly Line. And we—clinicians and patients—are the cogs in the machinery. Instead of ceding authority to physicians, we cede authority to government, administrators, and faceless algorithms. We more often treat a computer screen than a patient. And the doc isn't the boss, but neither is the rest of the health care team—nor the patient. We are ALL treated as commodities...raw materials in the factory.

"Taking the best aspects of 1.0 (deep sacred relationships, physician autonomy) and 2.0 (technology, evidence, teams, systems thinking), Health 3.0 restores the human relationship at the heart of healing. It bolsters that relationship with a team that revolves around the patient while supporting each other as fellow caregivers. What emerges is vastly greater than the sum of the parts.

Caregivers and patients have the time and space and support to develop deep relationships. Providers hold patients accountable for their health, while empowered patients hold providers accountable to be their guides and to know them—and treat them—as unique human beings. Our EHRs bind us and support us, rather than obstruct us. The promise of Big Data is translated to the unique patient in front of us. Our team provides the lift so everything doesn't fall on one set of shoulders anymore but on health coaches, nurses, social workers, lab techs, EVERYONE together. We are evidence-empowered but not evidence-enslaved. We are paid to keep people healthy, not to click boxes while trying to chase an ever-shrinking piece of the health care pie. Our administrators seek to grow the entire pie instead, for the benefit of ALL stakeholders."

You'll notice that insurance does not enter into Health 3.0, which, again, is concerned with what we buy and how we buy it, not with who assumes the financial risk.

A Pyramid of Health

Health care today is a tangled jumble of silos largely organized around medical technologies, not patients. This mess is exacerbated by economic models and information technology that further impair healing. A group of us[136] are trying to develop a structural model for an ecosystem that looks at health care as an asset rather than simply an expense or a revenue stream to be maximized. One of our key design points is that the ecosystem should be antifragile, a quality described by Nassim Nicholas Taleb in his book *Antifragile: Things That Gain from Disorder*. For those unfamiliar with Nassim Taleb's book, *Antifragile*, he introduces the book as follows:

"Some things benefit from shocks; they thrive and grow when exposed to volatility, randomness, disorder, and stressors and love adventure, risk, and uncertainty. Yet, despite the ubiquity of the phenomenon, there is no word for the exact opposite of fragile. Let us call it antifragile. Antifragility is beyond resilience or robustness. The resilient resists shocks and stays the same; the antifragile gets better."

Health care has been unique in that it uses technology as an excuse for costs to go up and productivity to go down. In Health 3.0, a properly organized health ecosystem can benefit from technology rather than helping fuel hyperinflation for all of us, while decreasing productivity and job satisfaction for clinicians.

We have used a pyramid to represent the developing ecosystem and show how various elements of health and health care interrelate. (The pyramid graphic below is the start of developing a North Star for how various elements of health and health care interrelate with each other.) Each layer represents a level of care or self-care*, and each has four facets, one for each side of the pyramid:

1. Optimal way to deliver health services
2. Optimal way to pay for care
3. Enabling technology for #1 & #2
4. Enabling government role for #1 & #2

Following a given layer (e.g., value-based primary care 3.0) shows how the four facets apply to that layer.

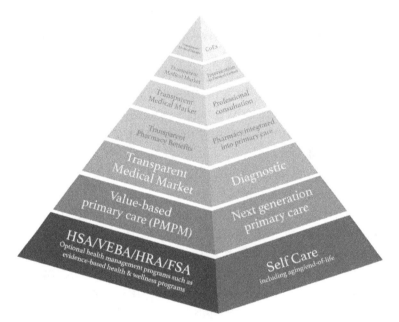

Figure 10. You can also explore an interactive graphic at healthrosetta.org/health30.

You want to spend as much of your life as possible in self-care at the bottom of the pyramid. When you have to move to higher layers, you want to move back down ASAP. You read the pyramid from the bottom and, at each layer, look at the four facets to ensure they are meeting your goals. Thus, you would see that the self-care layer is at the bottom. When you first access

---

* Note that self-care is necessary at all levels. However, it starts at the foundation. The pyramid is a holarchy. This just means it incorporates hierarchies that both transcend and include levels. They work like 3D concentric circles, rather than rungs on a ladder. Imagine looking at the pyramid from the top. You will have concentric boxes, with self-care transcending and including them all.

the health care system, next generation primary care is where you should start. In countries like Denmark and in the best value-based primary care organizations in the United States, over 90 percent of care can be addressed at this level, which includes things like behavioral health, interior work, health coaches, and physical therapy, all enabled by technology like secure messaging, remote monitoring, and other future advances.

Chapter 21 covers value-based primary care and focuses on high-cost individuals who consume most of the health care spending. For the majority of people who have simpler primary care needs, there are more streamlined, technology-enabled, and cost-effective methods of delivery. For example, Dr. Jay Parkinson has proposed what he calls "Primary Care 3.0" which is optimized for most people with simpler medical needs.[137]

If an issue can't be addressed in primary care, you move up to the diagnostic layer (e.g., lab tests) for deeper insight to rule in/out various issues. Then, if you need a prescription, you'd go to the next layer—pharmacy woven into primary care. Organizations such as ChenMed do this well. If a prescription isn't the answer, you proceed to the next layer for a "professional consultation" between the PCP and an objective specialist, that is, one who wouldn't be performing any necessary intervention or procedure. If an intervention is needed, you proceed to the next layer—intervention via focused care in a setting with deep experience in that particular intervention.

Jonathan Bush, Co-founder of Athenahealth, told me about his own knee surgery. Even the highest-volume knee surgeons in Boston, he found, do less than one-third of the procedures they could, spending the rest of their time doing marketing for their team. If they spent most of their time doing what they do best, they could drop their unit price.

Finally, the unfortunate few who have rare and highly complex conditions would go to a Center of Excellence for their condition (e.g., NIH and Mayo) at the top of the pyramid.

To reiterate, even when at higher levels of the pyramid, the goal is to move back down the pyramid as soon as possible.

As I developed this framework further, I was interested in getting specialists' feedback. Relatively speaking, I've spent more time with primary care physicians at the base of the pyramid. This framework reflects that the most advanced and successful value-based primary care organizations intuitively understand that two key issues drive costs and quality:

1. Fostering self-care and caregiving by nonprofessional loved ones is essential to optimizing healing and health.
2. Without a seasoned "ship's captain" (the primary care physician), rough medical seas cause patients to needlessly suffer from an uncoordinated health care system.

Specialists, like any group of humans, have many opinions, but I will share the feedback from Dr. Venu Julapalli on the framework (he has also been writing about the tenets of Health 3.0). [138] The following are Dr. Julapalli's comments, edited for length and clarity.

I am loving what you guys have come up with.

1. *It starts with self-care at the base. That's key. It underscores personal responsibility in health, which has been woefully neglected. At the same time, social determinants of health (SDoH) are right at the base, where they belong. I love the pyramid's government facet, letting it act as the market accelerator, not an overly active market participant without the ability to enable the most effective and efficient system.*
2. *It properly puts value-based primary care right near the base. As a specialist, I don't need to be near the base. I also need to have as few conflicts of interest as possible in my interactions with primary care.*
3. *It properly puts the specialist care in focused settings near the top (this position doesn't make them the most important, just the most focused). This is what Devi Shetty is executing in India and Cayman Islands—high-volume cardiovascular surgery by experts who love what they do, while dropping unit price ridiculously through streamlined operations and economies of scale.[139]*

4. It appropriately puts Centers of Excellence at the very top—go there for help with rare diagnoses, but keep it limited. We should also never forget the power of the engaged patient, who destroys the most expert doctors when love for life takes over. See this article as an example, "His Doctors Were Stumped. Then He Took Over."[140]

Overall, I love this pyramid framework. Conceptually, it's honoring much of what I've come to believe on health care, health, and healing. You're distilling what real-life experiences and data have shown works in health care.

Implications for providers and government

Major trends are making the care delivery elements of Health 3.0 a once-in-a-career opportunity (or threat). In the United States alone, experts expect $1 trillion of annual revenue to shift from one set of health care players to another over the next decade.[141] This is a byproduct of the transition to purchasing health care with accountability baked in. Here are some new realities providers and government entities must prepare to accommodate to thrive in a Health 3.0 world.

Health Care Provider Organizations

1. Convenience and accountability will be essential.

Various new primary care models such as onsite/near-site clinics and direct primary care have significantly expanded their scope of services (e.g., remote monitoring and health coaching). The top performers readily put their fees at risk (e.g., Vera Whole Health, PeakMed, and Iora Health). Medicare Advantage programs are taking off like wildfire, with the top performers delivering care far differently than in volume-driven models. If you're a health care provider, this is the future!

We expect Medicare Advantage to continue to grow and Medicaid Advantage to follow closely behind. This trend can't be dismissed as fringe when two early adopter organizations (Care-More and HealthCare Partners) were acquired for over $5 billion and there has been over $1.2 billion invested in next generation primary care models in the past few years.[142] Sadly, we hear of too many organizations trying to foolishly cling to fee-for-service and even enacting anti-competitive practices such as threatening doctors in their communities who don't refer to them (e.g., blocking data and patient flows).[143] Our message to you: Don't be scared; be brave. Be among the early organizations that figure out and master how to thrive in the inevitable future.

2. Millennials are moving in.

If you thought boomers were a big deal, millennials dwarf them and are transforming markets. This has already had a devastating impact on a local oligopolistic market (newspapers) similar to health care.[144] In another area of health, big food and big soda have had their worst earnings in decades caused by millennials adopting significantly different purchasing habits than their parents. The status quo in our current legacy health care system is nearly a perfect opposite of what millennials want and value. Organizations that think they're entitled to their patients' kids are in for a rude awakening. For most provider organizations, private employers are their most lucrative revenue stream, and millennials are already the biggest chunk of the workforce and expected to be 75 percent of the work-force in 10 years. As millennials wake up to the reality that they will be indentured servants to the health care system without change, expect their voices to be heard like never before. Health 3.0 is just what millennials want.

3. Destructive doctor relationships will destroy hospitals' success.

It's not just doctors who feel abused by the Health Care 2.0 system. However, the economic impact of burned-out doctors leaving in droves will stagger today's health care systems. The

ZDoggMD "Lose Yourself" anthem highlights the rising revolution of nurses, doctors, and clinicians who are saying "enough" and leaving for organizations focused on the Quadruple Aim.[145]

Government Entities

1. Be a smart buyer

It seems every local, state, and federal government is struggling with budget challenges—largely the result of health benefits being the second biggest expense after wages for many of them. As one public entity found, the best way to slash health care costs is to improve benefits (e.g., greatly improved access to value-based primary care).[146] Innovative new health care delivery organizations can serve a broader audience faster if governments are early adopters of higher-performing health benefits for their employees, thus freeing up public funds for the other social determinants of health. Further, it reduces the risk of public sector employees being enslaved by opioid use disorders.

2. Don't rob Peter to pay Paul

Government is in a unique position to improve public health and other social determinants of health—a position that is undermined by hyperinflating health benefits costs. Social and economic factors drive ~40 percent of health outcomes, compared with just ~20 percent for clinical care,[147] yet clinical care consumes far more financial resources. Forward thinking government leaders recognize the opportunity to cultivate what we call economic development 3.0, playing the high-performance health ecosystem card and creating enormous value for their constituents.[148] We all intuitively know that health care spending comes at the expense of other household spending. Economic Development 3.0 properly aligns limited public resources to improve social determinants of health and reduce working and middle-class wage stagnation.[149]

3. Don't accept in health care what you'd never accept elsewhere.

Imagine if local, state, and federal government contracts for road and highway construction did not insist on smooth connections between road sections. This is exactly what happens in health care: We pay trillions of taxpayer dollars to tax-exempt health care organizations, yet permit them to block implementation of many simple reporting processes and technologies, such as the simple exchange of vital patient information. Collectively, trillions have gone to health care organizations that lack even basic modern connectivity. Nowhere in our society are more lives in jeopardy. It's like military generals who are actively prevented from seeing the full battlefield.

Even worse from a public health perspective is the status quo's limited ability to facilitate two-way communication in crisis situations. We saw this recently with Zika, when health care providers using modern systems could rapidly respond to a threat while those using outdated approaches were left flat-footed. Modern, cloud-based electronic health records and other communication systems can rapidly identify and respond to public health threats, identifying regions and individuals at greatest risk.[150] Yet most organizations use outdated systems that require manual updates. This unnecessarily imperils the most vulnerable in society.

4. First, do no harm.

Sadly, many well-intentioned government efforts have unintended and damaging consequences, too often not understood until it's too late.[151] Government should stop blocking innovations that advance connectedness—stop dictating how technology companies share data and information—and focus instead on rewarding early adopters. Demand that the private sector deliver the right outcome, which is information flowing from all clinical data sources, and then let them get on with it. In short, government officials should adopt a Hippocratic Oath of their own.

I will conclude with a quote highlighting just how badly we need the major overhaul outlined in Health 3.0. Dr. Otis Brawley, chief medical officer for the American Cancer Society said, "I have seen enough to conclude that no incident of failure in American medicine should be dismissed as an aberration. Failure is the system."

Simply shifting who pays is just moving deck chairs on the Titanic. Metaphorically, we're all on the same ship.

Key Take-aways

- The health care system was built over the last 100+ years in response to random events ranging from wars to scientific breakthroughs, creating a tangled jumble of disconnected silos. A fresh reset rebuilding the health care system from the ground up is showing us the way toward the future.
- Eminence-based medicine, often free of evidence, gave way to evidence-enslaved medicine turning medicine into a transaction. Medicine-as-machine has been punishing to both clinicians and patients alike.
- Health 3.0 restores the human relationship at the heart of healing, bolstering relationships with a care team that revolves around the patient while supporting each other as fellow caregivers. What emerges is vastly greater than the sum of the parts.
- The most underutilized role of government is as a market accelerator of high-performing health benefits. For the most part, the 22 million public sector workers have health benefits that perpetuate the underperforming status quo health care system.

CHAPTER 18

ECONOMIC DEVELOPMENT 3.0: COMMUNITIES TAKE CENTER STAGE

"We're paying more for the privilege of getting sick and dying early. Once again, it makes no sense. And once again, no one in Washington is talking about how to fix it." – Michael Bloomberg

In his book *The Coming Jobs War*, Jim Clifton, Chairman of Gallup, makes a strong case that the United States is already in World War III. Unlike the previous wars, which dictated which countries would lead the world in prosperity as a function of property, the current war will dictate which communities will prosper by winning the lion's share of jobs. Civic leaders can and should seize this opportunity to reinvent their communities and build infrastructure.

The wisest leaders will shift how their communities think about economic development. It turns out that having a high-value health ecosystem is likely to be of greater benefit than a tax break. Conversely, communities with expensive health care have what amounts to a large health care tax that will push businesses away or, at a minimum, impair their bottom line and the well-being of their workforce.

The Post-Copernican View

Economic Development 1.0 was largely a function of geography: successful towns emerged near ocean and river ports or along transportation routes and capitalized on the need to shift goods and people efficiently.

Economic Development 2.0 has been largely a function of marketing: communities throw tax breaks at corporations to attract or retain them, without always considering the long-term effects. For example, building hospitals was perceived as an economic driver despite considerable evidence that adding capacity is actually an economic drainer after the "caffeine hit" of initial construction. This pre-Copernican view of health care puts hospitals and medical technology at the center of the health universe. The post-Copernican view puts individual and community well-being at the center of a properly functioning health ecosystem.

Economic Development 3.0 recognizes that all the tax breaks in the world are dwarfed by whether a community has a high-value or low-value health ecosystem. In Chapter 3, we explored the devastating impact health care has had on individuals and local economies as working and middle-class disposable income has increasingly vanished.

After payroll, health benefits are often the largest cost for most employers in both the public and private sectors. Just as manufacturers shift production to low-cost manufacturing centers, employers will be attracted to high-value health communities. For instance, IBM is making decisions on where to locate new technology centers based on the health care value equation.[152] Such decisions represent thousands of jobs for communities vying for growth opportunities.

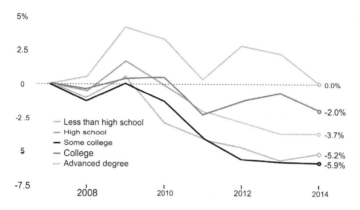

Cumulative percent change in real average hourly wages, by education, 2007-2014

Note : Sample based on all workes age 18-64.
Source: Epl analysis of Current Population Survey Outgoing Rotation Group microdata

Figure 11: 2014 Continues a 35-Year Trend of Broad-Based Wage Stagnation [153]

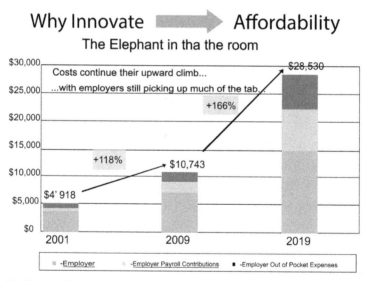

Figure 12: Per capita spending for IBM employees 2001, 2009 with projection for 2019.[154]

As we have seen, employers foot most of the health care tab[155] and are starting to flex their muscles. Thus, IBM shifted from thinking about health benefits as a soft benefit to seeing them as a major supply chain input that will impact its profitability. The company decided where to locate 4,000 new hires based on their analysis of where they would receive the best value from their health care expenditure. After looking at the graph below it's easy to understand why they picked Dubuque, Iowa.

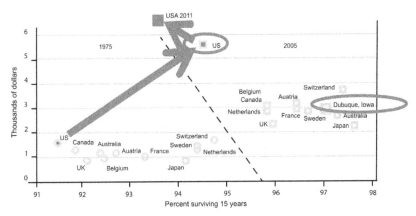

Figure 13: Per capita spending and longevity by country, 1975 to 2005, by locale.

Given the wide cost differentials, CFOs and CEOs are failing in their fiduciary responsibility if they do not move to modern health care delivery models that are proven to save money while maintaining or improving health outcomes and patient satisfaction. This is a scary prospect for communities that have high-cost health care with average outcomes.

Churchill was quoted as saying, "Healthy citizens are the greatest asset any country can have." It stands to reason that we should measure that asset. One could imagine a Community Well-being Balance Sheet as a leading economic indicator of prosperity. On the asset side of the ledger would be things like clean air, clean water, the number of high school/college graduates, community centers, and so on. On the liability side would be things like a Superfund site or outstanding hospital bonds.

We could also imagine something like a Gross Community Product: the collective revenues generated by local businesses subtracting out health care spending as a measure of people who are not able to contribute to community well-being. Forward-looking economists are developing new economic indicators to better reflect the health of communities.

Taxation Without Representation

Jeff Brenner, MD, founder and long-time executive director of the Camden Coalition of Healthcare Providers, currently senior vice president of Integrated Health and Social Services at UnitedHealthcare Community & State, and a 2013 MacArthur Genius Grant recipient, spoke about health care as a tax on a community[156] that the residents didn't get to vote on—a tax that negatively affects a community's competitiveness. He points to a "giant hospital bond market" that brought too many hospital beds online. An empty hospital bed, says Brenner, is the most dangerous thing in America.

"In the center of New Jersey… a couple years ago, they built two… $1 billion hospitals, 10 miles apart, very close to Princeton. One is called Capital Health, and the other is Princeton Medical Center. I don't remember anyone in New Jersey voting to build two brand-new hospitals. But we are all going to be paying for that the rest of our lives. We'll pay for it in increased rates for health insurance. And, boy, you better worry if you go to one of those emergency rooms, because the chances of being admitted to the hospital when there are empty beds upstairs… are… much, much higher than when all the beds are full – whether there's medical necessity or you need it or not. I'd be very worried if you live in Princeton that there are now two $1 billion hospitals waiting to be filled by you."

Every health system CEO I've spoken with agrees with health policy expert Paul Keckley, PhD, that there is at least a 40 percent over-capacity of hospital beds,[157] and some communities are still building. A recent Harvard School of Public Health study of 195 hospital closings found that the closures had no discernible impact on outcomes.[158] In fact, in countries that have shifted from a "sick care" model to a model that is focused on health and well-being, more than half of hospital beds were no longer needed. This is something to celebrate. While we have to be mindful of short-term impacts on individuals working in these facilities, there are higher and better uses for most of these people (e.g., health coaches and investments in health-enhancing infrastructure), especially at a time when there is full employment.

Even though many health systems are tax-exempt nonprofits, perverse incentives have created a dynamic where revenue growth has become a central objective. In reality, tax-exempt nonprofits make up 70 percent of the most profitable hospitals,[159] perhaps because their boards are typically made up of business leaders who reflexively view revenue growth as the goal when it should be community well-being and addressing major issues such as the opioid crisis. Hospital executives also realize it's easier to justify enormous compensation packages if their institution is generating massive revenue increases every year. As Axios reported, "Large not-for-profit hospital systems now resemble and act like Fortune 500 companies instead of the charities they were often built as. They consequently hold immense financial and political power."

In contrast, forward-looking nonprofits focus on long-term economic sustainability and their mission to serve as stewards of community health. With all of the changes in health care, it's just a matter of time before more enlightened boards fundamentally rethink their mission to emphasize the 80 percent of nonclinical factors that contribute to health and well-being.

Closing a Hospital Opens Other Doors

One of the most respected health care leaders in the country, David Feinberg, MD, CEO of the renowned Geisinger Health System, believes his "job ultimately is to close every one of our hospitals," in order to take care of individuals at home, work, and school.

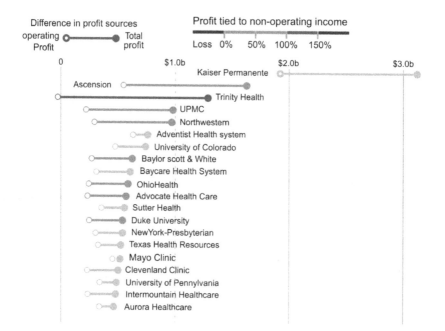

Figure 14: Operating and total profit by health system[160]

As overcapacity gives way to hospitals optimized for the health of communities, those communities will realize a bonus: hospitals are often in locations with high real estate values. According to David Friend, chief transformation officer at the consulting firm BDO in Boston, "a hospital could be worth more dead than alive."[161] Hospitals are often in city centers with great access to transit. Wide hallways, thick walls, and high ceilings make them easy to convert to housing. Communities have repurposed hospitals to a wide variety of uses, from low-income senior housing to health and wellness centers to office space.[162]

Being alarmed by a hospital closing is understandable. However, experience shows that this can open great opportunities while rarely affecting health outcomes. An analogy from military bases is enlightening: the closing of Philadelphia's naval shipyard was bitterly fought, yet now the repurposed naval yard is the most dynamic development in Philadelphia.[163]

Rethinking Economic Development

Here are some examples of how forward-looking civic leaders are embracing Economic Development 3.0.

- Freeing up financial resources formerly dedicated to unnecessary and harmful clinical procedures allowed Rosen Hotels & Resorts to invest heavily in its community; the result was a reduction in crime of 67 percent and a doubling of high school graduation rates. The Rosen case study outlines how a single private employer pulled this off, but any employer—public or private, large or small, corporate or government—can do the same. In New Jersey, public and private unions joined with a Democratic Party-dominated legislature and then-Governor Christie to find common ground around improving health benefits to lower health care costs.
- Communities have found that "Shop Local" programs lead to more dollars circulating in the local economy. Health care is a fundamentally local interaction, yet the value creators (nurses and doctors) receive less than 25 percent of every dollar spent, with a much larger percentage going to bloated administration or overhead, fraud, waste, and abuse that robs communities. Municipalities as employers and trendsetters are increasingly contracting directly for health services in order to keep money in the community. For example, directly contracting with locally owned surgery and imaging centers[164] rather than with health chains owned by out-of-towners is increasingly common. The potential to recirculate dollars with locally-owned health care provider organizations is enormous.
- Mayors and economic development directors are catalyzing locally controlled health insurance pools referred to as "captives" where multiple organizations pool risk. Think of it as the health insurance equivalent of the Green Bay Packers where they are owned by a community with local control but have the ability to tap into national-scale contracts, reinsurance and technology.

- As large employers themselves, municipalities are getting much smarter about how they purchase health benefits, using the components outlined in the Health Rosetta blueprint. With respected organizations, such as PwC, acknowledging that more than half of health care spending is waste, it's logical that financially-strapped municipalities are rethinking their approach, as described in the Kirkland, Washington, and Milwaukee case studies.

- The historically adversarial relationship between school boards and teacher unions has hurt communities throughout the country. Proactive city leaders recognize healthy schools are one of the most important factors in attracting and retaining citizens. In an announcement about a new teachers' union agreement in a school district that covers one of the wealthiest areas of the country, one major accomplishment cited was that "teachers will see protection from rising health care costs," largely as a result of school district concessions. While this is laudable, the smartest districts and unions are realizing they're on the same side when it comes to health care costs and can collaborate to slay the health care cost beast, as they did in Pittsburgh. (See the Pittsburgh case study for more).

Sooner rather than later, we can expect other developments along the same 3.0 spectrum. Cities will incorporate true health needs into master planning and review building permit applications with a deep understanding that health care is a supply-driven market. The more supply there is, the more demand will increase, with little regard for value and community well-being. Approving more health care build-out virtually guarantees a massive burden on local citizens.

Forward-looking city attorneys and state attorneys general will challenge the non-compete agreements that doctors have signed as being against the public interest. In particular, primary care physicians (PCPs) are foundational to a more effective health system. Though they were ostensibly money losers in the waning fee-for-service industry, PCPs can refer more than $8 million per year in revenue to the rest of a health care system. As a result, health systems have gobbled them up to protect their flank and create captive referral channels, insisting on anti-competitive deals that harm a well-functioning health ecosystem.

The #1 cause of personal bankruptcy is health care costs,[165] recently exacerbated by an opioid crisis largely inflicted on society by a failed health system. This has a profound impact on the economic vitality of neighborhoods and communities, dragging them into a downward spiral caused by overtreatment. Millennials will push back hard as they have in so many other sectors like banking and marriage. Indeed, we saw in Chapter 6 that staying on the current health care path will mean that millennials will spend over half their lifetime earnings on health care. There will be riots in the street before that happens.

I believe in the enormous potential of community-driven change from the bottom up. Central governments have largely reached the limits of what they can achieve. Increasingly, community-level change is where the action is.

Key Take-aways

- Economic Development 3.0 recognizes that all the tax breaks in the world are dwarfed by whether a community has a high-value or low-value health ecosystem.
- Closing a hospital can open doors to myriad economic benefits to a community. Transforming hospitals and hospital beds to higher and better purposes is a sign of progress.
- "Shop Local" comes to health care providing an unprecedented economic stimulus opportunity.

CHAPTER 19

MAYORS MUST LEAD CITIES OUT OF THE OPIOID CRISIS

"Cities can basically do anything except declare war and sign treaties, and that gives you a whole lot of room to rip and run" — New Orleans mayor Mitch Landrieu

Health doesn't start at the hospital or with a pill. Health starts at home. That puts mayors and school superintendents/principals—who, along with other local leaders, are tackling society's toughest challenges today—on the frontlines of the opioid crisis.

Cities and counties have already filed hundreds of lawsuits against drug manufacturers to recover money invested in combating the opioid crisis,[166] including:

- costs of implementing opioid prevention and treatment programs
- health insurance payments for municipal employees, retirees, and their families
- costs incurred by first responders to overdose calls
- court and crime-related expenses
- other social costs of addiction, including expenses for employee Narcan training.

Cities are also seeking reimbursement for future costs, including some that historically have not been considered municipal services, such as rehabilitation for those with opioid use disorders and counseling services for their families. Perhaps the most difficult to quantify are the indirect costs, such as the children who become wards of the state after losing one or more parents to an overdose, the emotional toll the crisis takes on emergency responders, and the lost economic productivity.

It may take these lawsuits years to be resolved, so wise civic leaders aren't waiting around. Instead, they are turning the can-do spirit that is the hallmark of cities and towns on upstream preventive strategies. Since the opioid crisis is symptomatic of the larger health care dysfunction, the adage, "a crisis is a terrible thing to waste," applies.

Key Strategies for Civic Leaders

Beyond the horrifying human cost of the opioid crisis, the national financial cost is staggering, with the latest estimate being over $500 billion.[167] While that figure is hard to get your arms around, local leaders can easily see the money extracted from their communities each year, as we spelled out in Chapter 16, to make it more comprehensible.

Using estimates from Chapter 16 about the amount of funds that get extracted from a local community's economy, the potential for recapturing that lost economic benefit should be appealing for mayors. Using a rough estimate of $5,000 per person (half of the $10,000 total per capita spend) in health care spending being extracted from a local economy, a city of 100,000 people sees $500 million leave their economy each year. Imagine if those dollars were recycled in a local economy. These extracted dollars include a mix of fraud and what economists call "rent seeking" behavior—an extraction of value from others without making any contribution to productivity—common in PPO network and PBM pricing outlined earlier, just to name a few.

We often limit "shop local" thinking to retail and food, but it is just as applicable in health care. One could argue it's even more so, as health care delivery is fundamentally about a local relationship between a clinician and a patient. The opioid crisis is just a window into the damage inflicted by under-performing elements of the health care system. The following are the key strategies for civic leaders to pursue:

Use Your Bully Pulpit

Virtually every employer in America, including public-sector entities, has funded the opioid crisis. After all, the vast majority of those enslaved by opioid use disorders are working-age people or their dependents. Unlike past public health crises where a primarily government-led effort has been effective, the opioid crisis can't be solved without employers fundamentally changing their approach to health benefits. Thus, mayors and other civic leaders must enlist the business leaders who employ the bulk of the community.

In many realms, the public sector has been a great second-wave customer after an industry has proven the commercial market viability of a product or service. New and better building practices are an example; private developers were the early adopters of LEED-certified buildings, followed by many cities and states that required new public-sector buildings to follow LEED standards. Public-sector employers as market accelerators may be the biggest missed opportunity in health policy. A side benefit is that it can take health care policy debates from ideology-based to evidence-based at the local level, where ideological divides often break down.

In the third most watched TED talk ever, "How Great Leaders Inspire Action," Simon Sinek recommends that you "start with why," that is, that you start by sharing the higher purpose of organizational change. It's understandable that both employees and employers are skeptical of benefits changes; they have been conditioned for twenty years to accept paying more for less every year; they typically won't understand that the best way to slash health care costs is to *improve* benefits. The combination of explaining their personal benefit *and* the broader community benefit is the path to transforming initial resistance to change. Share the Pittsburgh schools and the Rosen Hotels case studies with them to demonstrate how not squandering health care dollars translates into better benefits and greatly improved opportunities for kids.

Stop Fraud

Fraud is so much more pervasive than most of us (including myself) have guessed. If your community is like others, up to 10 percent of your health care spending is leaving your community because of fraud.[168] A modest investment in payment integrity technology and claims audits will quickly shed light on the magnitude of your local problem.

If your insurance company or claims processor balks at providing complete access to full claims data, you can be quite confident they have something to hide. It's time to change who you are working with. As outlined in Chapter 26, anyone managing a health benefits plan has a legal duty that prohibits turning a blind eye to fraud.

Address Substance Abuse

Wise employers realize that the costs of not addressing substance use disorders is high. Seventy-five percent of adults with substance use disorders are in the workforce and the yearly economic impact may be more than $442 billion dollars. Workplaces bear a large portion of those costs through absenteeism, increased health care expenses, and lost productivity. When the substance being abused is pain medication, workers cost employers more than three times the health care costs of the average worker.[169] According to the National Survey on Drug Use and Health, one of the main drivers of this financial burden is the fact that only 10 percent of those suffering receive any type of specialized treatment. Many things contribute to this treatment gap, including lack of screening in the health care system, lack of access or ability to pay for care, and fear of shame or discrimination. In fact, a recent study indicated that twenty four percent of those with this disease do not seek treatment because they do not want their friends, family, and co-workers to know about it.[170]

Employers are paying the price for untreated substance use in three areas; increased absenteeism/lower productivity, increased job turnover/retraining costs, and increased health care utilization. To quantify these costs, the nonprofit Shatterproof, the National Safety Council, and the independent social research organization NORC developed the Substance Use Cost Calculator; they found the costs range from $2,600 per employee in agriculture to more than $13,000 per employee in the communications sector.

Rebuild Primary Care in Your Community

Put simply, the opioid crisis can't be solved without a rebuilt primary care system that gets rid of the fundamentally flawed fee-for-service model. There have been well-intentioned efforts to improve primary care. A "patient-centered medical home" (PCMH) is a common approach that has laudable elements. Already overburdened primary care doctors who are spending an hour or two on bureaucracy for every hour of patient time have understandably taken a "check the box" approach to PCMH to get some modest bonus payment that goes to cover compliance with new requirements. The sad fact is that the rise of the PCMH movement paralleled the rising opioid crisis. The point isn't that the PCMH was the cause of the crisis but that putting wings on a car doesn't make it an airplane.

Smart leaders realize that substance use disorders (SUD) are a chronic condition, not unlike many other chronic conditions that are best addressed in a proper primary care setting. Primary care physicians can now be board certified in addiction treatment, so they can serve their community's needs. The monthly fee to treat and manage the SUD is much more cost-effective than the financial and emotional ripple effect of being enslaved with a SUD, costs that are felt by families, employers, and communities.[171]

When unburdened by insurance bureaucracy and volume-based fee-for-service payment models, primary care is the foundation of a properly functioning health care system. Functioning primary care, a relative rarity in the U.S. today, addresses three key areas:

1. More than 90 percent of the issues that drive people into the health care system can be fully addressed when a primary care doctor has time to do more than order unnecessary prescriptions, referrals, and tests.
2. It's estimated that 80 percent of health care spending is a byproduct of lifestyle choices. These issues are almost impossible to address in the less than 30 minutes a typical person spends with their doctor throughout the year in today's typical primary care model. Full primary care consists of a team that includes health coaches, nutrition experts, and others with the time, empathy, and expertise to reverse common lifestyle-related conditions such as Type II diabetes. Long-term chronic conditions can also lead to mental health issues, which are commonly treated with non-evidence-based opioids and benzodiazepines, leading to further exacerbation of the conditions.
3. Primary care physicians (PCP) are a vital ally when dealing with medical conditions beyond the scope of a primary care practice. A PCP with sufficient time is a trusted advisor who can ensure that individuals avoid misdiagnosis and over-treatment in low-value settings. There is no one more trusted by patients than a non-conflicted PCP with the time to fully explain treatment options, and this relationship often heads off unnecessary surgeries and tests.

Value-based primary care organizations, such as Vera Whole Health, guarantee their results and have been certified by the rigorous Validation Institute.[172] In contrast, many health benefit plans use an array of Band-Aids for undermined primary care, such as urgent care, retail clinics, primary care telehealth, care coordination/management from insurance carriers that are unnecessary and wasteful when proper primary care is in place. Seattle and Denver are two examples where primary care is being rebuilt brick by brick to the point that most employers in these two metropolitan areas have access to value-based primary care clinics.

Making Health Local Again

This book focuses on non-legislative strategies since the politics of health care are fraught with pitfalls. As we know, the best way to perpetuate the status quo is to politicize a topic—and nothing is easier to politicize than health care. Having said that, we have an opportunity where interests overlap: The right likes local control and the left likes expanding access to care.

Even countries that are perceived to have a nationally controlled health care system, such as Sweden, have more local control than the United States. The national government sets some overarching principles. However, at the regional level, responsibility for financing and providing health care is decentralized to county councils typically representing less than 500,000 people—sometimes much less. At the local level, municipalities are responsible for maintaining citizens' immediate environments, such as water supply and social welfare services. Recently, post-discharge care for the disabled and elderly and long-term care for psychiatric patients were decentralized to the local municipalities in Sweden. Local councils have considerable freedom in deciding how care should be planned and delivered, with room for wide regional variations.

Just as it took a while for the built infrastructure to be transformed by LEED, a steady stream of grassroots innovation that proves itself before being replicated is how we will transform health care in the United States. The following are efforts to make health local again, drawing on promising health care innovations:

- Localized captive insurance plans: Most companies under 50-100 employees aren't comfortable being self-insured, thus losing the freedom to design a smart benefits plan. Localized captive insurance plans allow multiple organizations to pool together to form their own insurance entity. Mayors are catalyzing locale-specific captives to gain more control and keep money in their communities. Others are supporting legislation allowing for portable benefits untethered to one's job – a particularly acute need for the millions who are freelancers, gig economy workers, temporary workers and contractors.

- Due to the agreement struck between unions and the Governor Christie administration, New Jersey is on a path to have the largest statewide coverage of value-based primary care. After the pilot phase, it will allow locally owned and controlled primary care clinics to tap into state funds to serve local communities.

- A little-known element of the recent tax legislation is a provision called the Investment in Opportunity Act, which allows the estimated $2 trillion in capital gains sitting on the sidelines to be invested in distressed communities representing over 50 million Americans by deferring capital gains taxes. It's early in the process, but some investing groups are coming together to invest in things like local grocery stores in underserved areas and community-owned clinics. A good analogy for this is how the Green Bay Packers are community-owned, yet also benefit from an affiliated national entity.

- The Accountable Communities of Health (ACH) is a program from the Centers for Medicare & Medicaid that allows regional groups analogous to Sweden's county councils to keep savings in their region when they achieve successes, such as reducing hospitalizations. In the status quo model, if a county hospital is able to reduce Medicaid hospitalizations, the financial reward stays at the state capital. With ACHs, saved money can be reinvested into other health-supporting initiatives such as community centers, public safety, walkability, etc.—all at the discretion of the local organization managing the ACH.

- There are recent ongoing efforts to create Federal legislation establishing Community Shared Savings Accounts in Medicaid. Drafts of this legislation would establish grants from the federal government for states to provide data to communities to identify the top 20 Medicaid cost areas. Communities could choose to implement programs seeking to improve the health of the Medicaid Beneficiaries and reduce costs. When communities validated that their efforts resulted in cost savings, a large percentage of those savings would be allocated to the community shared savings account to be overseen by a local board. The funds could be used for initiatives that improve the community's health status.

- Hospital districts have been a fixture for decades, especially in rural areas. Historically, they have been just as dependent on the perverse incentives of fee-for-service payment models. Emerging in places such as Pennsylvania are All-payer Global Budgets[173] that remove the incentive to fill hospital beds to stay financially afloat. If they can achieve 50 percent reduction in hospitalizations as other communities and countries have, this frees resources to invest in other health outcome drivers, such as clean water, better food, treatment programs, education, and health-promoting jobs, including community health workers and health coaches.

Key Take-aways

- Mayors must use their bully pulpit to convene business leaders in their community to solve a massive crisis. It will be impossible to solve the opioid crisis without active engagement by employers in a community since it is their health benefits that are funding and fueling the over-prescribing of opioids leading to downstream opioid use disorders.
- Fraudulent health claims payments both drain resources out of local economies, but they also enable opioid diversion. Mayors should lead by example, ensuring that an independent claims audit and payment integrity review is done for city employees.
- Rebuilding primary care in communities is foundational to solving both the opioid crisis and the larger squandering of economic resources by a wasteful health care system that extracts dollars out of local economies.

- There's no more important role for mayors than ensuring the safety and well-being of their community. Re-localizing health risk management from distant out-of-town health insurance companies to locally rooted and accountable organizations is vital to creating healthy communities.

CASE STUDY

RURAL COUNTY GOES FROM HIGHEST TO LOWEST RATE OF OPIOID DEATHS IN TWO YEARS

Faced with startlingly high rates of opioid-related deaths, leaders in four rural counties in Northern California mobilized to combat the problem. Health care providers and the public health department quickly formed the Northern Sierra Opioid Safety Coalition in January 2016. Demonstrating the power of a comprehensive approach, the county with the highest rate of opioid-related deaths had none in all of 2017.

James Wilson, a health education coordinator with Plumas County, and his colleagues were the first to notice the spike in death certificates listing opioid overdose as the cause of death. Along with public health officials from Plumas, Modoc, Lassen, and Sierra counties, law enforcement, social service nonprofits, hospital leaders, and county elected officials also played pivotal roles in the regional coalition.

The coalition received a grant from the California Health Care Foundation (CHCF) to accelerate their efforts. Rather than mandating solutions, CHCF designs the grants to provide local leaders with the flexibility to define their unique situation. So, the coalition was able to address the epidemic from multiple angles, including:

- adopting safer prescribing practices
- expanding access to effective addiction treatment
- implementing community approaches to overdose prevention
- coordinating communication between historical silos, such as emergency departments and primary care providers.

The national opioid epidemic has hit remote, rural areas like the Northern Sierra particularly hard. Geographic isolation and limited medical resources have exacerbated the situation, leaving both law enforcement and small local hospitals struggling to keep up. With a goal of curbing the growing number of opioid-related addiction and deaths in the four counties and expanding access to treatment for those already enslaved by opioid use disorders, the coalition focused on three areas: promote safer prescribing, widen treatment options for addiction, and increase access to naloxone, which can counteract the effects of an opioid overdose.

"Detailing" is a technique pharmaceutical companies use to educate a physician about a vendor's products, including opioids, in hopes that the physician will prescribe them more often. Taking a page out of the drug company's playbook, the coalition hired a pharmacist to do "academic detailing" to educate physicians about safe prescribing and demonstrate the link between pain management and addiction. It's working.

In Plumas County, according to data provided by Wilson, the volume of opioid prescriptions has declined by nearly a third. In the second quarter of 2011, there were 1,234 opioid prescriptions per 1,000 people. In the fourth quarter of 2017, that number was 867 per 1,000 people. For those already facing addiction, the coalition pursued the gold standard for treating opioid use disorders – medication-assisted treatment (MAT). Previously, the nearest MAT provider was a 90-minute drive away, in large part because physicians were reluctant to invite addicted individuals into their clinics. The academic detailing, informed by prescribing data for specific physicians, allowed doctors to see that they were already treating addicted patients; they just didn't look like stereotypical "addicts." Today, there are six physicians in the area able to provide MAT.

Since September 2016, the coalition has distributed 500 naloxone doses in the four counties and recorded 18 overdose reversals. Data from the California Department of Public Health demonstrates a dramatic decline in opioid deaths in Plumas County. In 2014, the county had 20.52 opioid-related deaths per 100,000 residents, compared to the state's overall rate of 4.92. In 2015, the county's opioid death rate was 31.3 per 100,000, compared to the state's rate of 4.73. By 2016, however, the most current records available show there were no opioid-related deaths in Plumas. This is progress anyone would brag about, but coalition leaders understand that a problem this systemic requires sustained investment. Even at the reduced level, opioid prescriptions are still higher than evidence-based best practices would dictate.

As they look to the future, the coalition will expand primary prevention, safe drug disposal, academic detailing, clean syringe access, and more harm reduction strategies while maintaining the programs already started. The Northern Sierra counties show how adapting proven approaches to local conditions can turn the tide on the opioid crisis. No one is more committed to local communities than local citizens and leaders. The silver lining to the opioid crisis is a reminder of how even systemic problems can be successfully tackled, whether it's the opioid epidemic or any other problem where status quo approaches have failed.

CHAPTER 20

MAKING SURE OPIOID MITIGATION PLANS MITIGATE THE RIGHT THINGS

"It's clear they're not going to be part of the solution unless we drag them to the table." — *Jonathan Blanton*

Dozens of cities and counties and virtually every state have filed or are in the process of filing lawsuits against the opioid supply chain—opioid makers, drug distributors, pharmacy benefits managers, retail pharmacies, and insurance carriers. These communities argue that these organizations have externalized the full damages caused by opioids to local communities, employers, and states. In other words, the opioid supply chain has profited while communities have paid the massive price from the fallout.

The situation mirrors the $300+ billion tobacco litigation settlement. Mike Moore, the former Mississippi Attorney General (AG), was the first AG to file a tobacco suit and ultimately became a leader in combining dozens of other suits into one. Having personally been touched by the opioid crisis, Moore is once again helping orchestrate myriad cases on this new front. Their plan is to apply the lessons from the massive tobacco settlement, in particular how the settlement can be a catalyst for a long-term fix—not simply holding liable parties accountable for their externalized costs.

Typically, the person who falls into opioid addiction is, at the start, a gainfully employed individual with a pain problem, often a back pain problem. As outlined in Chapter 1, they get a prescription for an opioid from their overworked doctor, become addicted, have addiction-related problems at work, lose their job, go on Medicaid, and may end up using street opioids such as heroin or fentanyl after they can no longer afford prescriptions. This, in turn, leads to a host of other issues, such as Hepatitis C and incarceration. It can transpire remarkably fast, leaving local communities and states to pick up the tab.

An effective mitigation plan requires that we fully understand the underlying problems, so that the plan is up to the challenge it faces. Early attempts at solutions have been inadequate or worse, creating other problems. The goal of this chapter is to inform those involved in settlement discussions on what is most likely to solve the immediate problem while also addressing upstream issues to prevent a recurrence.

The Opioid Mitigation Plan

Naturally, the primary goal of any mitigation plan is to solve the problem. However, we are also mindful that the opioid crisis is emblematic of health care's broader dysfunction and believe that this is an opportunity to fix the root causes of the broader dysfunction. For example, many of the factors that drive pharmaceutical prices sky-high come from elsewhere in the supply chain—not the drug makers. Thus, we expect some of the new market norms imposed in the mitigation plan to be embraced by pharmaceutical companies.

The following is a prioritized list of opioid mitigation items, an outline of the mitigation strategy, and some additional background to help further understand the situation.

Value-based primary care for those suffering from opioid use disorders should be covered for life (similar to asbestos victims).

Core problem solved: As with asbestos, dealing with opioid addiction is a lifelong chronic medical condition. The biggest inappropriate prescriber has been volume-driven, fee-for-service primary care that has become the norm over the last 20 years—prescribing behavior driven by pharmaceutical rep training of doctors who were told that opioid medications weren't addictive. This has been compounded by bad incentives that drive overly short primary care visits and well-intentioned but flawed patient satisfaction ratings.

Additional background: This greatly increases the avoidance of inappropriate opioid use. Leaders in primary care, such as Bluegrass Family Wellness, not only provide great value-based primary care (VBPC), their physicians have also obtained board certification in addiction medicine; unlike traditional fee-for-service primary care, they have adequate time with patients to provide comprehensive care, including wellness advice and other counseling. For an additional monthly fee, they also provide medication-assisted treatment, which is currently viewed as the best long-term treatment approach for opioid use disorders. By helping reinvigorate primary care (via value-based primary care), this approach solves what is arguably the single biggest failing of the U.S. health care system. It's critical that primary care vouchers should be set up to seamlessly transfer between Medicaid, private insurance, and Medicare. It is common for those in the working class to move on and off Medicaid and it's vital to not force doctor change. This also helps the recipients become more employable, lowering the burden on the employer for any substance use disorder (SUD) medical needs.

Pharmaceutical companies must fully disclose compensation to those in drug supply chain, including pricing standardization.

Core problem solved: Compensation between drug manufacturers, distributors, PBMs, pharmacies, and insurance companies is at least as impactful as compensation physicians receive from drug manufacturers (which already requires disclosure). Disclosure should include those in the financial and physical chain of custody for all drugs to help prevent future occurrences.

Note: Drug makers are still allowed to set their own pricing under this proposal; however, it must be standard across the board. Likewise, it is okay to have volume discounts as long as they are equally applied. This is consistent with the Fair Trade for Health Care outlined in Chapter 12.

Additional background: Physicians must already publicly report compensation for speaking, consulting, and other financial arrangements with pharmaceutical manufacturers. Pharmaceutical companies feel they're over the barrel, particularly by PBMs, to provide rebates and keep underlying costs as opaque as possible. Drug makers also spend inordinate amounts of time negotiating deals with various members of the supply chain, so a standard, transparent pricing program would be a welcomed relief. Manufactured drugs can win on merits rather than compensation schemes. It is important that standardized pricing be a part of this; otherwise, kickbacks can be buried in pricing. Press exposés into "King of Pain"[174] and "Wizard of Oz"[175] marketing schemes give a small glimpse into how insidious compensation and marketing schemes can be.

Every form of media should be used to wake up America to systemic failure and to destigmatize addiction.

Core problem solved: Many Americans believe that the opioid crisis is caused by lazy, weak-minded people. It's critical that they come to understand the truth—that the cause is systemic rather than individual, that stigmatization of addicts is a major barrier to treatment and thus employment, and that appropriate care will relieve the economy of a huge burden.

Additional background: Reaching different people will require different kinds of approaches, media and technology in light of the diversity of those impacted.

Combine medical, pharmacy, and workers' compensation claims.

Core problem solved: Inappropriate prescriptions are easier to flag when data is combined. Currently, medical, pharmacy, and workers' comp claims are typically separate.

Additional background: A common database can be a valuable source of R&D for drug manufacturers on how their medications are being used—not to mention the potential to avoid fraud, waste, and abuse.

Publicly report on prescribing volumes by physician and organization.

Core problem solved: This requires reporting of oversubscribers at the individual and organization level. When this is coupled with combining medical, pharmacy, and workers' comp claims, it can also get at overprescribing at the procedural level.

Additional background: Much addiction starts with surgeries and other areas of care beyond primary care settings, so reporting can highlight where there is overuse. For example, reporting can improve care by minimizing or eliminating opioids for anesthesia, driving adoption of approaches perfected in Belgium that are being successfully used in the United States. Further, Johns Hopkins's Dr. Marty Makary, founded the Center for Opioid Research and Education to reduce post-surgical prescribing variation by procedure (see http://www.solvethecrisis.org). Even within a respected institution such as Johns Hopkins, prescribing patterns vary widely from one physician to another for the same surgery with the same patient health status.

Eliminate direct-to-consumer pharmaceutical marketing.

Core problem solved: Americans have been trained to seek a quick fix for every medical need, impairing physicians' freedom to properly prescribe based on medical needs versus advertising-induced patient demand.

Additional background: When combined with physician compensation predicated on patient satisfaction scores, demands by patients put severe pressure on physicians to prescribe medications they wouldn't otherwise be inclined to prescribe. Note that this would include all forms of advertising, such as broadcast, Internet, print, and in-office ads.

Reform Workers' Compensation.

Core problem solved: A focus on the treatment of the whole person (aka BioPsychoSocial-Spiritual treatment model) is slowly but surely replacing the BioMedical model and an overreliance on some<u>body</u> (e.g., a physician) or some<u>thing</u> (e.g., a pill) to treat injuries. In practice, this means workers' comp payers encouraging—and paying—for alternative treatments that otherwise would be overlooked or even denied.

Additional background: Factory owners are discovering that their own shop floors are home to drug rings—with the company itself as the supplier. Prescription opioids, and the corresponding medications to treat the side effects (constipation, sleep disorders, over-sedation, increased anxiety, dry mouth, etc.), have been used in workers' comp care as long as it has in general health care. However, workers' comp became more acutely aware of this inappropriate polypharmacy (using multiple drugs to treat the same medical issue) sooner than other payers.

While some noticed the issue as early as 2003, the industry, as a whole, started to notice in 2009 as Medicare Set Asides began to include future prescription drug treatment over the injured worker's lifetime. The oversimplified calculation—current treatment plan multiplied by the rated life expectancy—created exorbitantly priced lifetime care that often included long-term use of prescription drugs (such as opioids and benzodiazepines) that were never meant to be used in that way.

Since that time, various tactics have been employed, through state regulations and industry innovations, to reduce the use of these drugs. Examples include evidence-based treatment guidelines, drug formularies, utilization review, management peer review, morphine equivalent dosage and day supply thresholds, pharmacy benefit manager controls, provider networks, claims settlement strategies, predictive analytics, and stakeholder education.

As a result, opioid utilization has decreased steadily since a peak in 2014. However, there is also a growing awareness that removing medications while ignoring methods to develop coping skills and resiliency is not only short-sighted, but suboptimal for the well-being of the injured worker and the finances of whomever pays for treatment. While there is a role for opioids in the treatment of acute and even chronic pain, their scope as it relates to medical appropriateness and risk versus benefit calculations is much smaller than is currently supposed. Hence, the ever-increasing advocacy for alternative means of pain management.

This includes modalities such as yoga, mindfulness, biofeedback, physical therapy, acupuncture, cognitive behavioral therapy, better nutrition, proper sleep, hygiene, smoking cessation, life coaches, and a number of other approaches to pain management (including medical marijuana) that up to now have been largely denied by payers.

In other words, the focus should be on creating individualized treatment plans that seek out the most beneficial modalities with the least negative repercussions. This takes more effort—by the payer, provider, and patient—and might even cost slightly more up-front, but ultimately results in better outcomes and lower costs. While progress has been and is being made, much more is needed. In some ways, workers' comp is leading the way.

Implement consumer media/education on appropriate methods of addressing pain and risk from opioids.

Core problem solved: Consumers have been trained by incessant advertising that there is a pill to solve every issue. Creative media letting people know how they're being gamed can change mindsets. Curriculum that is age-appropriate can be made freely available on the web to education publishers and through sites such as Khan Academy.

Additional background: Through grants and investments, problem-solvers can draw on a wide array of creative media vehicles from traditional film to Snapchat snippets that can educate and influence people in entertaining ways.

Informed consent on opioid prescriptions.

Core problem solved: Most patients unwittingly follow doctor's orders and have no idea that drugs such as OxyContin and Vicodin are highly addictive. Informed consent and shared decision making should be standard protocol in all care settings.

Additional background: Outreach resources need to get baked into the clinical workflow of care provider tools such as EHRs.

Require certification to prescribe opioids with accompanying medical education/detailing.

Core problem solved: Many people enter the health care system with some form of pain. Opioids are the blunt instrument to address this, even though there's a more appropriate modality in most circumstances. For various opioid "on-ramps" (e.g., joint pain, mental health, etc.), the focus should be on PCPs, but also include relevant specialists such as rheumatologists.

Additional background: Big pharma marketing tactics can be used for good purposes. Instead of drug manufacturers influencing doctors in a strategy called detailing, "academic detailing" will update physicians on the latest science on the best methods of treatment, which typically don't include opioids, as detailed in Chapter 1.

The pharma industry and supply chain must adopt certified, value-based primary care for their employees.

Core problem solved: Employers, without meaning to, nonetheless drove the opioid crisis by paying for "drive-by" primary care and poorly handled care for mental illness and musculoskeletal pain leading to overuse of drugs.

Additional background: The pharma industry can help accelerate / bootstrap widespread high-quality primary care that is opioid-resistant.

Require full chain of custody reporting/auditing for both the physical pills and payment for opioids.

Core problem solved: In many industries, the physical and financial chain of custody is a foundational component for ensuring safety, preventing fraud or abuse, and sustaining properly functioning markets. Applying principles from sectors such as food safety, banking, and other financial transactions and organizations (e.g., market making and clearinghouse activities) would lay the proper foundation to prevent the next pharmaceutical crisis, or at least catch it before it reaches epidemic levels. For example, it would enable accurate reporting and disclosure at many points in the supply chain from manufacture to prescription, particularly around disclosure of financial payments and prescribing volume.

Additional background: Much of the infrastructure for this already exists across the pharmacy supply chain, but a review of current processes and capabilities, as well as state and federal laws, would identify gaps that should be addressed. Audits and public reporting for both physical custody and financial transactions is critical to prevent future crises, as gaps in either will leave more opportunity for future abusive behavior. Finally, this would create a more integrated supply chain, reducing operating costs and opening the door for new lines of business for various supply chain players.

Highlight and fund successes around social determinants of health (sDoH), celebrating cities that are fostering improved sDoH through a series of contests.

Core problem solved: A lack of focus on the social determinants of health has created more fertile ground for the opioid crisis to fester.

Additional background: Call it a tax write-off, call it community rebuilding… As Sam Quinones wrote in *Dreamland: The True Tale of America's Opiate Epidemic,* the ultimate antidote is rebuilt communities, in which the social fabric and the economy are shaped around healthy behaviors. This could probably be paid for with philanthropic dollars from big pharma.

Key Take-aways

- When an industry such as tobacco externalizes the costs of its products, it is accountable for those costs. The lessons from the tobacco settlement will inform the optimal opioid settlement.
- If industry practices aren't reformed, the opioid crisis will be repeated. Already, the benzos crisis is at the level the opioid crisis was at ten years ago. For example, the flow of money through the health insurance companies and pharmacy benefits managers is just as influential as drug maker payments to physicians, which are already transparently reported.
- Media and education is critical to destigmatizing those enslaved by opioid use disorders. If we stigmatized people receiving treatment for diabetes or heart disease, they would also avoid getting treatment.

- When primary care is badly undermined, it creates fertile ground for overprescribing drugs such as opioids. When primary care is trapped within volume-centric health systems designed to maximize fee-for-service revenue, it fuels non-evidence-based treatments such as opioids or surgeries for back pain.

Part IV

Restoring Hope, Health, & Well-being in Our Communities

This is the vision, roadmap, and how-to portion of the book. Political tumult in the United States and around the world has laid bare the profound failings of the status quo. As we saw in Part I, the effects of health care's dysfunction play a far bigger role in the unrest than many realize. It's time for a reset. In this section, we describe the mindset shift that is driving dramatic results in companies, unions, not-for-profits, and all types of communities: small towns and large cities, rural and urban.

Mayors and municipal governments are on the front lines, solving problems that seem intractable at the national level but are highly solvable at the local level. The Health Rosetta blueprint represents the work of the best minds in health care benefits, public health, and economic development, including specific guidance on how leaders are going upstream to stop the opioid crisis at its source. Many have had many years of sustained success. This section also compares status quo approaches with proven best practices.

The Health Rosetta evolves nearly every day as evidence and ideas are shared in this open source community. Like the Rosetta Stone, the Health Rosetta is the path to deciphering health care's hieroglyphics.

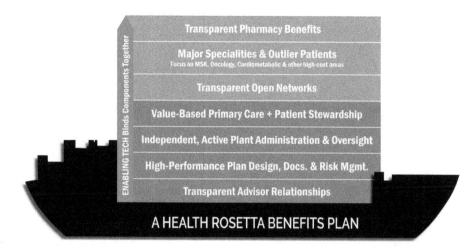

In many ways, today's health plans are like ports before the standard shipping container. That is, ports operated in a haphazard manner as a legacy of hundreds of years of small modifications. Wise health care purchasers have rethought from the ground up, how a modern health benefits plan should be structured. Just as the cost to ship dropped dramatically and safety was improved, wise health care purchasers are seeing tremendous savings and safety improvements.

CHAPTER 21

VALUE-BASED PRIMARY CARE

"The physician who teaches people to sustain their health is the superior physician. The physician who waits to treat people until after their health is lost is considered to be inferior. This is like waiting until one's family is starving to begin to plant seeds in the garden." – Unknown

What is Value-based Primary Care?

Value-based primary care (VBPC) is an umbrella term for various delivery models that involve direct financial relationships between individuals or employers and primary care practitioners (PCPs) *outside* of the traditional fee-for-service (FFS) insurance model, typically managed by your plan administrator. Value-based primary care offers patients, physicians, and purchasers an alternative to traditional FFS payment arrangements, in which physicians are reimbursed according to the volume of services they provide, regardless of quality. VBPC has matured as health care purchasing shifts from volume- to value-based payment models.

Value is defined as the ratio of quality to cost. Value increases as the quality of the care increases or the cost of care decreases.

In the United States, there are two primary models for VBPC, though this space is evolving rapidly with much more differentiation emerging:

- Direct primary care (DPC), in which care is offered directly to individuals, plan administrators, and employer in a range of practice models from solo practitioners to national organizations
- Onsite/near-site clinics fully or partially dedicated to the workforce of a specific employer

How Does It Work?

Providers of VBPC typically charge a monthly, quarterly, or annual membership fee, which covers all or most primary care services including acute and preventive care. The fee is paid out of an individual's own pocket, by a sponsoring organization such as an employer or union, or by a health plan offering commercial or government programs, such as a Medicare Advantage plan. Most commonly, the practice has been devoted to the particular sponsoring entity (e.g., a near-site clinic for employers/unions or a Medicare Advantage-based clinic devoted to seniors), but models that serve multiple clients are maturing.

The flawed incentive structure of FFS demands very short primary care appointments, which often drive referrals to unnecessary high-margin services such as scans and specialists and result in an overreliance on prescriptions. The reduced overhead from eliminating FFS billing also allows VBPC practices to offer a more proactive care model that can lead to significant reductions in downstream costs.

Why Should You Support It?

VBPC aligns your interests with primary care providers, which can improve health outcomes and significantly lower costs for your employees and members. Health outcomes are improved by shifting the focus from reactive, episodic care to a continuous care relationship, population health strategies such as preventive and chronic care, optimized specialty care referral channels, and care management.

The VBPC model also delivers a substantially better experience for patients, often in one or more of the following ways:

- More time with their provider
- Same day appointments
- Short or no wait times in the office
- Better technology, e.g., email, texting, video chats, and other digital-based interactions
- 24/7 coverage by a professional with access to their electronic health record
- Far more coordinated care

VBPC also improves provider experience and professional satisfaction, which, in turn, is known to improve the quality of care.

What Are the Key Elements to Look for in a VBPC Provider?

1. Quality Reporting

Clinical quality measures (e.g., What percentage of patients were vaccinated in line with standard schedules? Required hospitalization? Received domestic violence screening?) are reported in appropriate detail to:

- The individual patient
- The purchaser
- A community health information exchange (HIE), where available

2. Shared Decision Making

PCPs use established communication techniques to ensure patients are educated and engaged in making decisions about their own care, being respectful of preferences, ethics, and economic concerns. Coordinating efforts with employers and health plans, PCPs clarify and validate health information about patient conditions, rights, and available options.

3. Care Coordination

PCPs actively coordinate care with specialists and ancillary providers, ensuring post-hospital and post-surgical follow-up. Care coordination should not be predicated or dependent on all providers sharing a common electronic health record (EHR). Employers and plans should exert leverage on all nonconnected providers to share information via an HIE.

4. Population Health Management

Management of chronic conditions is proactive, aggressive, and team-based, using patient advocates, care manager nurses, and personal health assistants/coaches. Care is facilitated by using patient registries, either embedded in the EHR or through collaboration with the HIE.

Preventive services include evidence-based screenings (specifically excluding those known to be harmful or of questionable value) and active pursuit of both childhood and adult vaccinations according to current recommendations from the Advisory Committee on Immunization Practices of the Centers for Disease Control and Prevention.

5. Value-based Payment Models

Compensation models reward physicians on a nonvolume basis, such as straight salary, per member per month fees, or the overall number of patients for which they are responsible. Purchasers should look for a portion of VBPC provider compensation being dependent on value, as determined by some combination of quality metrics, patient experience scores, and resource stewardship. The general nature of the compensation model should be transparent to help inform the purchaser's selection of providers.

6. Patient Experience

Standard methods are used to measure patient experience and engagement. Patient advisory panels are incorporated in the practice to offer guidance about service functions and assure a patient-centered orientation. Purchasers should expect to see aggregated experience scores as one measure of quality.

7. Evidence-based Medical Care

The practice is grounded in evidence-based medicine—as demonstrated to purchasers through transparency of clinical process and outcomes measures, as well as provider education and collaboration—that respects patients' insurance coverage or financial status, personal preferences, and ethics.

8. Physical Therapy Embedded within the Practice

The trigger for many people entering the health care system is a pain symptom. Physical therapy woven into the triage and primary care process ensures the proper care pathway for issues commonly mistreated with opioids and non-evidence-based orthopedic procedures.

9. Ease of Access to Care and Care Information

A patient portal is available to access personal health records and facilitate asynchronous communication between patients and providers. A patient is not expected to make an office visit unless physical presence is necessary for quality of care. The practice collects data on standard access metrics and shares them with a patient advisory panel and the health care purchaser, and provides complaint resolution and follow-up. Patients have 24/7 telephone access to a health care professional with immediate access to the patient's, thus reducing unnecessary ER use.

10. *Clinical Pharmacy and Mental Health Embedded within the Practice*

The practice provides clinical pharmacy support for patients with complicated drug regimens and those requiring additional support for drug-related concerns, including resources to help patients unable to afford prescribed pharmaceutical treatments. Mental health services for common issues (typically depression and anxiety) that can be managed on an ambulatory basis are readily and conveniently available through the primary care office.

11. *Physician Loyalty*

At all times and in all matters, including testing, referrals, hospitalizations, and all care outside the office, physicians and other providers in the PCP practice align with the patient's care interests and personal economics. Physicians strive to deliver the highest quality at the most reasonable cost and put patient interests above others.

12. *Referral Patterns*

VBPC clinics should take an active role in referring patients to high-value specialists and facilities.

What Challenges Can You Expect?

1. *Administrative Challenges*

Your broker, consultant, carrier, or TPA may be unable or unwilling to help you evaluate the appropriateness of VBPC for your health plan.

2. *Employee Education*

Employees in established primary care practices may be unwilling to switch to one using a VBPC model—at least initially. Inertia, comfort with current providers, and lack of awareness of their current care quality are all impediments. Being able to demonstrate both financial and nonfinancial benefits to them is key, as is making clear that they are not being forced to see a "company doctor." The need for frequent, clear communication with employees and dependents can't be overemphasized.

3. Care Dislocation

Having large numbers of people switch primary care physicians can be challenging, especially when physicians in the receiving practice may be overwhelmed by the sudden increase in a short period. Talk with the new physicians to understand their capacity and access issues. Don't wait for your employees and their families to complain.

4. Criteria for Choosing a Practice

Practices may market themselves as low-cost providers, but primary care should never be purchased solely on cost. Expect to spend more on high-quality primary care in return for downstream savings and other benefits (e.g., increased productivity and employee satisfaction) that will more than cover the increased costs. Choose primary care based on patient service, demonstrated clinical quality metrics, and demonstrated attention to stewardship of your dollar.

5. Care Coordination

Current providers and health systems may warn that VBPC encourages care fragmentation and loss of coordination, no longer a tenable argument in today's digital age. Insist on the adoption of a health information exchange and other technology to overcome this barrier.

6. Slow Migration to the New VBPC Model

People are much more willing to change PCPs when they get to meet the doctor beforehand. If possible, arrange for your new PCPs to visit with employees at your workplace. Also, arrange tours of the new practice location. Employers willing to provide strong incentives to try out the new primary care model will achieve much higher adoption rates.

7. Obfuscation to Preserve Status Quo

Physicians who aren't forward-looking may fall back on "fear, uncertainty, and doubt" tactics meant to freeze progress. As stewards of your organizations' and employees' hard-earned money, you must choose whether to protect your own bottom line or that of your vendor.

What Action Steps Can You Take?

Ask your broker, consultant, insurance carrier, or TPA if they are currently working with or have experience with VBPC practices.

Encourage your broker, consultant, carrier, or TPA to find, interpret, and share reliable cost and quality data from primary care groups competing for your business.

Consider comparing primary care groups through a structured and disciplined RFP process. Also consider modifying your benefits plan to provide incentives for employees and their families to try a VBPC practice.

Visit a local VBPC practice and see for yourself.

Additional Resources

Please visit healthrosetta.org/health-rosetta for ongoing updates, including lists of value-based primary care organizations, case studies, best practices, toolkits, and more.

CHAPTER 22

TRANSPARENT OPEN NETWORKS

"The single most important ingredient in the recipe for success is transparency because transparency builds trust." – Denise Morrison

What is a Transparent Open Network?

A transparent open network (TON) offers purchasers such as employers and unions fair and fully transparent pricing for medical services/procedures ranging from specific treatments (e.g., knee replacement or colonoscopies) to specific conditions (e.g., diabetes or kidney disease). Services and procedures are typically bundled, meaning there is just one bill for all the services received for a specific treatment or condition that includes multiple providers and sometimes multiple settings. Another dimension of transparency is that the market is open to any provider who has sufficiently high-quality indicators and charges fair prices.

A TON offers employers an alternative to traditional fee-for-service (FFS) payment models, in which individual services are listed on itemized billing statements from multiple sources.

How Does It Work?

Providers (typically independent imaging centers, specialty hospitals, ambulatory surgery, and some forward-looking hospitals) supply up-front pricing at significantly reduced rates in exchange for increased volume, quick pay, reduced friction, and avoiding claims/collections problems—all factors that allow providers to net a similar amount to standard insurance billing while charging less.

Providers contract directly with an employer or third-party to offer services outside of a typical payment and network structure. In exchange for significantly reduced rates, employers encourage plan members to use these providers, typically by waiving all of the individual's costs including copays, coinsurance, and deductibles.

How Does Reference-based Pricing Fit in?

Reference Based Pricing (RBP), also commonly known as Cost Plus Pricing, offers self-insured plans a defined benefit structure with more economical reimbursement levels. These are based on various pricing data sets, most notably Medicare, and are designed to be fair and reasonable to providers. RBP vendors offer nationwide coverage and countless employers have had great success with them. Some people believe they put employees at risk for balance billing but, in reality, the RBP vendors address this in their service contract. (And of course, we know employees are already at tremendous financial risk with status quo plans, high deductibles, confusing billing, and more.) It can also be seen as confrontational, because the employer is essentially telling the provider what they are willing to pay as opposed to the provider setting the price.

The reality is very few issues crop up and they are overwhelmingly addressed in a simple manner. In most cases, the RBP discussion opens a broader conversation and starting point for a TON, often leading to direct contracting. RBP vendors commonly handle the transition for a high-volume provider organization to a direct contract that they facilitate.

Why Should You Support It?

Unlike FFS, which allows for wildly variable, opaque pricing free from market forces, which can incentivize providers to offer unnecessary services, TON benefits providers, employers, and employees. Providers get access to individuals whose employers offer quick pay and reduced hassles, while employers get access to bundled, transparent rates at prices typically 30 to 50 percent lower than typical *network* discount prices (and even more off of chargemaster prices). Employees get access to a new benefit that offers medical services and procedures without financial penalties in the form of copays and deductibles. In short, providers get easier administration and certainty, employers get great prices, and patients get the care they need at no additional cost.

What Are the Key Elements to Look for?

Transparency

It's not possible for employers to measure the value of their health care dollar without access to pricing and quality information. The same information is needed by employees if they are expected to seek high-value care. At a minimum, all medical services and procedures should be available at fair, honest, and up-front prices, making health care services as straightforward as other products and services we buy. Quality information should also be readily available for employers and employees alike.

Bundled Payment

Bundled payment for a specific treatment allows employers to trade endless, confusing, itemized bills for just one bill covering the hospital, surgeon, anesthesia, equipment, etc. For treatment across a specific condition there is just one bill for all physician visits, diagnostics, and care management.

Shared Risk

Medicare has long required providers to share risk under three different "global" periods (zero-day postoperative, 10-day postoperative, and 90-day postoperative) by refusing to pay for mistakes, complications, and re-admissions. A TON brings that practice to private health plans.

Efficient Administration

Typical claims administration is filled with inefficiencies: slow payment cycles, prior authorization, network requirements, complicated payment models, employee cost sharing, etc. For a TON to work, employers must make it easy for employees to access care, offer quick pay to providers (typically five days or less), eliminate barriers like copays and deductibles, and often remove administrative requirements such as prior authorization. It's important to remember that the goal of this model is to simultaneously lower employer costs, reduce costs and eliminate hassles for providers, and provide a true benefit to employees and members.

Employee Education

Models that encourage the use of specific providers for specific treatments are often a new idea for employees and their families. They need to understand that TON is *not* like HMO models, which were often associated with denied care, long wait times, and poor customer service. The message needs to be simple, clear, intriguing, and very short, preferably one sentence: *Don't forget, if you need medical care, we have a group of the highest-quality providers you can see, and choosing this won't cost you anything out of pocket.*

Ease of Use

Health care has always been confusing, frustrating, and very often scary. A TON should be effortless. Consider offering concierge-style customer service, which gives your employees easy access to the humans and resources they need, including hassle-free appointment scheduling, medical records transfer, and both web and mobile access. These services can also create comfort for your employees around sensitive health issues they don't want to discuss with you or your internal benefits manager.

How Can You Ensure Quality?

An effective TON functions best in tandem with a value-based primary care model and use of shared decision-making tools to avoid overtreatment and radiation exposure from unnecessary scans. Any high-quality provider should be participating in all applicable quality reporting whether they are a health system, ambulatory surgery center, imaging center, or independent physician practice. Here are some resources that can help ensure that the providers you use are, in fact, of the highest quality.

- *HealthInsight* is a private, nonprofit, community-based organization dedicated to improving health and health care. They offer a free ranking tool for hospitals nationwide.
- *The National Quality Forum* (NQF) is a nonprofit, nonpartisan, membership-based organization that works to catalyze improvements in health care. They offer access to a huge library of evidence-based quality measures.
- *Hospital Compare* is a government website that allows you to find and compare quality information for more than 4,000 Medicare-certified hospitals across the country.
- *The Leapfrog Hospital Survey* is the gold standard for comparing hospitals' performance on national, professionally endorsed standards of safety, quality, and efficiency that are most relevant to consumers and purchasers of care.

What Challenges Can You Expect?

1. Administrative Challenges

Your broker, consultant, carrier, or TPA may be unable or unwilling to provide transparent specialty care and the administration to execute a TON.

2. Provider Reluctance

It is common for the large health systems you currently use to push back on requests for price and quality transparency.

3. Complex Implementation

The process can be quite cumbersome and drawn out should you decide to go it alone. You might consider using a third party to help streamline the process.

4. Employee Education

TON models require continued messaging and clear, easy-to-understand action steps.

5. Data Sharing

It could be difficult to obtain pricing and quality information from your current broker, consultant, carrier, or TPA. Since it is your spend, you have a right to this information.

6. Data Analytics

Traditional claims analysis software programs and services are often limited in scope and not designed to provide clarity or actionable insight.

7. Confusion about Price Transparency Tools

Many price transparency tools (e.g., Castlight) provide information on insurance PPO network pricing, but they don't remove the hassles and costs for either providers or individuals related to claims, copays, etc.

8. Obfuscation to Preserve Status Quo

Your current providers who aren't forward-looking are likely to use common "fear, uncertainty, and doubt" tactics meant to freeze progress. As stewards of your organizations' and employees' hard-earned money, you must choose whether to protect your bottom line or that of your vendor.

What Action Steps Can You Take?

Ask your broker, consultant, carrier or TPA if they participate in any transparency initiatives.

Encourage your broker, consultant, carrier, or TPA to make cost and quality data available to both you and your employees.

Consider modifying your benefits plan to provide incentives for employees and their families to access care from transparent providers.

Visit a local hospital or surgery center to discuss or consider tapping a third-party TON vendor in your region that may expand to serve your employees.

Additional Resources

Please go to healthrosetta.org/health-rosetta for ongoing updates, including lists of TON organizations, case studies, best practices, toolkits, and more.

CASE STUDY
ENOVATION CONTROLS

A Small Oklahoma Manufacturer Removes 97% of Pricing Failure

When you think of innovative organizations that provide a best-of-breed health benefits package and spend far less than peer organizations, you wouldn't necessarily think of small manufacturers in Oklahoma, where as much as 75 percent of the population doesn't have an established primary care relationship. Yet Enovation Controls, a provider of products and services for engine-driven equipment management and control solutions with about 600 employees, has managed to save approximately $4,000 per covered life each year by working with a transparent open network (TON).

A TON puts together a network of the highest-value providers for different kinds of care and gives self-insured employers a set of fair and fully transparent pricing—typically a bundled price—for medical services/procedures ranging from a specific treatment (e.g., knee replacement or coronary stent) to a specific condition (e.g., diabetes or kidney disease) across multiple providers, and sometimes, multiple settings.

Enovation Controls chose The Zero Card to manage their TON. They achieved a 70 percent participation rate among eligible plan members, focusing on high-cost services like surgeries and imaging. Justin Bray, Enovation's vice president for organizational effectiveness and human resources, attributes the high rate to two primary factors.

1. **Communications** – During the rollout of the TON, Enovation shared their current health care costs with employees, along with the consequences for the company and each individual. They then compared those costs with the costs of care under specific scenarios with TON. The message: We've found a better way. Most people were shocked by the vast price disparity and that lower-priced providers often delivered the highest quality, in part because these doctors perform a given procedure more frequently, improving with repetition and letting them operate efficiently with fewer errors and expensive complications.

2. **Ease of Use** – Employees have access to a single app or phone number that directs them to network providers where they can get care with zero out-of-pocket costs. Instead of dealing with a mountain of bills and paperwork following the procedure, they receive a thank you survey to ensure the experience went well. As Bray explained, this is particularly critical as surgeries and imaging are some of the highest-cost items they have to cover. Because of the focus on higher-cost items, Enovation has achieved well over 90 percent of projected savings, even with less than 100 percent participation. The calculation of those potential savings compared the historic "allowable" amount from the company's claims history with a true market amount through the TON network, that is, what a provider would accept if you showed up with a bag of cash for a bundled procedure such as a total knee replacement.

The savings over historical allowable amounts from their traditional PPO network ranged from 21.92 percent to 81.28 percent, with an average of 59.23 percent.

Here's an example of a line item for one procedure for one employee.

"Spinal fusion except cervical without major complications"

Historic allowed amount	$129,138
TON network	$38,000
Savings	$91,138

Bray shared what this meant to one employee who came up to him at a high school football game to say thank you. This person had recently had expensive surgery and didn't have to pay a dime out of pocket—no bills, no explanations of benefits, no anything. On a $30,000 salary, the maximum allowable out-of-pocket cost of $2,500 under the previous health plan would have been a financial disaster, the employee said.

Enovation Controls Employee Monthly Premium Costs

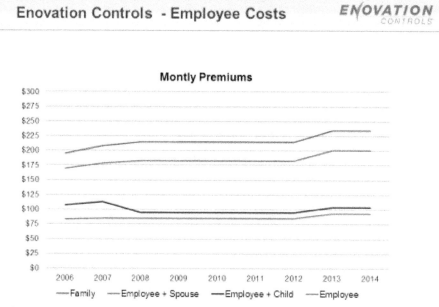

Figure 15. Summary information provided by Enovation Controls.

Like every other health care purchaser, Enovation Controls knows that tackling high-cost procedures is central to slaying the health care cost beast. Its TON program even extends to items like complex cardiac and neurosurgical procedures, for which employees have access to the same centers of excellence as large employers, such as Mayo Clinic. Whether the Mayo Clinic or a local surgery center, high-quality providers are happy to provide a deep discount in return for more business, less hassle, and avoiding claims processing and collections processes. Once the procedure is complete, the provider gets paid within 5 days for the full bundled price.

Plus, the bundled prices frequently carry warranties, meaning post-surgical complications within 60 to 90 days are addressed at no charge—another bonus for employers.

Using data from Mercer, Enovation Controls estimates that they save $2 million on health care every year, compared with peer manufacturing organizations. For a relatively small company, this is a highly meaningful amount of money, which it has been able to reallocate to increased R&D. While companies in their sector typically spend four percent of annual revenues on R&D, Enovation spends nine percent, helping it stay ahead of the competition and attract and retain the best engineers.

Enovation Controls Per Capita Spending

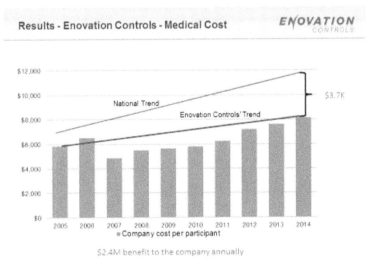

Figure 16. Summary information provided by Enovation Controls.

241

When a small manufacturer with few dedicated resources can pull this off, it begs the question why every employer or union isn't doing the same. Smart employers like Enovation Controls demonstrate that it's possible even in a state with some of the highest obesity rates and overall health care costs. Since a new primary care model or TON can be implemented at any point in a benefits cycle, there's no need to wait.

CHAPTER 23

CONCIERGE-STYLE EMPLOYEE CUSTOMER SERVICE

If you trust Google more than your doctor, then maybe it's time to switch doctors." – Jadelr and Cristina Cordova

What Is Concierge-Style Employee Customer Service?

Concierge customer service addresses a substantial challenge that exists for health consumers today—namely that the benefit and health care ecosystems are enormously complex and costly to understand and navigate. Current trends toward high deductible plan design only amplify the time and money required by you and your employees to make more intelligent decisions. Proliferation of solutions that address one or two discrete consumer needs, such as scheduling, price transparency, or finding a provider, still leave the individual to synthesize information across disparate sources, often during a serious health crisis.

Concierge service is the conductor that harmonizes much of this discord and fragmentation, providing one point of interaction and distilling complex information down to actionable guidance.

How Does It Work?

Concierge services are available as a subscription benefit for employees in value-based reimbursement contexts. They come in different forms. At one extreme, there are progressive concierge services driven entirely by algorithms that offer guidance based on machine learning. At the other extreme, there are more traditional, high-touch, one-on-one concierge services. In the middle, there are hybrid models built on "human-driven" technology, offering a balance between live support and technology-driven solutions. Members can speak with live support or, if they prefer, navigate through an intuitive mobile or web interface.

Members can access a broad spectrum of support services in a single interaction or series of interactions. Specifically, the concierge can provide:

- Triage
- Explanations of appropriate and available care
- Selection of plan-approved locations
- Help scheduling care
- Cost estimates
- Advocacy for claims and billing questions

The key to an effective concierge experience is integration of information so employees have hassle-free access to simple and actionable guidance on any issue when they need it. To make this work, concierge services are ingesting more and more data to improve the value of their support, tapping into information about plan design, provider networks, real-time benefit consumption (e.g., deductible and out-of-pocket status), individual preferences, and cost and quality data.

Why Should You Support It?

Concierge services integrate and coordinate a vast array of fragmented solutions into one location, enhancing engagement and optimizing benefit use at lower costs.

Employees who understand the implications of their consumption decisions are empowered to more intelligently navigate the care system. This means they can avoid unnecessary expense. As consumers use concierge services frequently and stretch their health care dollars further, risk-bearing employers, insurers, and providers can accrue savings as well.

Many programs that employers have invested significant dollars in, like the small number of appropriate and effective workplace wellness programs, require years to deliver return on investment. Concierge services can deliver savings in year one by guiding your employees away from unnecessary high-cost care.

Concierge support at "critical moments" builds lasting loyalty among employees. Helping individuals understand their benefits and access the optimal care in a time of need capitalizes on powerful teachable moments to build awareness of how individuals can be smarter health care consumers on an everyday basis. Finally, concierge services can be implemented off cycle and introduced successfully in advance of open enrollment as a benefit that can help employees select the best plan for their circumstances. Many times, employees are more comfortable selecting higher deductible plans when they know they will have concierge support as they navigate the care system.

What are The Key Elements to Look for?

1. Network Directories

Robust concierge offerings integrate the appropriate provider directories to accommodate complex network designs, including centers of excellence, onsite care clinics, or high-quality networks. The concierge directs members to the highest tier in-network providers for the highest level of care at the lowest cost, avoiding low-value providers and the costs incurred as a result.

2. Price Transparency

Concierge services should help employees prepare both clinically and financially for appointments by explaining the cost of an encounter upfront.

3. Scheduling Capability

Exceptional concierge services go a step beyond and schedule care on the employee's behalf.

4. Understanding of the Individual Consumer

A hallmark of true concierge care is a deep understanding of the individual consumer—including preferences and health profiles—so that care itineraries are personalized and thus more likely to be followed.

How Can You Ensure Quality?

Before contracting with a concierge service—and when considering renewal—ask to see documentation of the following:

- **Engagement** – What portion of a concierge service's potential population is using the service and how frequently?
- **User satisfaction** – What is the Net Promoter Score associated with the concierge service? In other words, would members recommend it to a friend or loved one?
- **Savings** – What savings has the concierge service delivered for members to date?
- **Marketing support** – What steps does the service take to reinforce member awareness on a regular basis through marketing campaigns, webinars, incentives, etc.?

What Challenges Can You Expect?

1. Employee Education

Such models will require continuing messaging and clear, easy-to-understand action steps so that concierge services remain top-of-mind for employees when the need arises.

2. Data Sharing

It could be difficult for your concierge service to obtain pricing and quality information from local providers. Since it is your spend, you have a right to this information, and experienced concierges can overcome this barrier.

What Action Steps Can You Take?

Ask your broker, consultant, insurer, or TPA if they are familiar with concierge offerings and how they may benefit your health plan.

Evaluate the return on investment from your current benefits toolbox by assessing member utilization rates and savings. If employees aren't using the tools, they may be overly complex, incomplete, or fragmented.

Survey your employees' aptitude for understanding and efficiently navigating the benefits landscape. Do they have an easily accessible resource to guide them through the lifecycle of a health care episode? Are they able to use the appropriate resources at the appropriate time to make educated decisions at the point of service?

Additional Resources

Please go to healthrosetta.org/health-rosetta for ongoing updates, including lists of concierge customer service organizations, case studies, best practices, toolkits, and more.

CHAPTER 24

HIGH-VALUE, TRANSPARENT TPA

"A lack of transparency results in distrust and a deep sense of insecurity." – *Dalai Lama*

What is a High-Value, Transparent TPA?

Third-party administrators (TPAs) charge a monthly fee for paying claims and performing other administrative functions for self-insured employers' health plans. Administrative services organizations (ASOs) associated with large carriers perform similar functions.* However, a high-value, transparent TPA does more. It can transform health care benefits from a black-box line item that increases by double digits each year to a cost center that you can actively manage and control. The value is evident in dramatic cost reductions that can be as high as 40-50 percent.

As a result, more and more employers are looking beyond large, well-known insurance carriers and have, instead, embraced local, regional, or national TPAs to help them translate health care costs into known, actionable components.

---

* ASOs often refer to themselves as TPAs. For clarity, when I refer to TPAs, I'm referring to TPAs independent of large insurance companies. See Chapter 13 for a more complete explanation of the distinction between ASO and independent TPA.

How Does It Work?

Employers can choose whether to bundle specific services they want in their monthly fee, depending on how engaged they want to be. Most high-value TPAs offer employers a range of provider networks (or no network at all, if you prefer) and integrate other innovative, third-party solutions to tackle costs and/or improve member experience.

A high-value TPA researches the cost of health care services and recommends actions that employers can take to save money. The following chart, adapted from the Colorado Business Group on Health, illustrates how astute employers and their high-value TPA partners measure and act on their employee's health care data.

Care Type	Measure	Action
Chronic care	Incidence/rate of chronic illness, gaps in care, and variation in physician practice patterns	Increase access to and payment for high-value primary care; educate about, remind, and encourage patient adherence
Episodic/outpatient services	Unwarranted variation in pricing for generally undifferentiated services; over-utilization of procedures driven by specialists and inappropriate demand	Increase employee education and decision support; pay for and encourage second opinions
Tertiary care	Variation in cost/outcomes by hospital service line	Designate centers of excellence; expose quality data by hospital and service line

Why Should You Support It?

Employers using high-value, transparent TPAs can actively reduce unnecessary health care costs while boosting the quality of health care services, thus improving the health and experience of employees and their families. If you are self-insured and purchasing care using, in part, your employees' money, this should be the minimum fulfillment of your fiduciary responsibilities.

Good health not only improves morale and productivity, it enables you to spend less on health care and more on growing your business. And employers have a unique ability to lead the change in health care that is so critical for the economy.

Sticking with a big-name insurance carrier through an ASO may feel like an easy, safe way to provide health benefits to your employees, which it certainly can be. However, employers who choose to partner with a high-value, transparent TPA typically do so because they are sick of convoluted rules, data that isn't actionable or accessible, opaque provider contracts, constant administrative runaround, and paying unknown and irrational amounts in exchange for services that don't add value.

A high-value TPA enables high-value primary care, concierge customer service, transparent open networks, centers of excellence, and more. In sum, it enables control over health care costs. It's a critical step toward fixing health care in America.

What Are the Key Elements to Look for?

1. Health Care Cost Transparency

Cost transparency means that the TPA helps you see how much you should be paying (the fair market price) for distinct services and the price variance between providers. Cost transparency can be achieved by standardizing prices according to regional benchmarks or Medicare pricing.

2. Quality Data

Having access to reliable data on hospital and/or physician performance is a necessary starting point for developing centers of excellence and other approaches to managing high-cost procedures. While quality data are still imperfect in health care, they are a necessary and valuable starting point for directing care. A high-value TPA will be adept at navigating the various sources of data.

3. Utilization Data

Health care utilization numbers without relevant benchmarks are useless. A high-value TPA will focus on appropriate use of services at the right time, right price, and right location or care setting. It does this by tackling underuse of primary and secondary preventive services for people with chronic conditions and use of low-value episodic treatments that are often not medically necessary.

For example, the following list of low-value services was developed by the Oregon Health Council. A high-value TPA can help reduce use of these wasteful services.

- Outpatient upper endoscopy
- Outpatient MRI, CT, and PET screening
- Spine surgery for pain
- Orthopedic joint procedures
- PTCA
- Stents
- CABG surgery
- Nuclear cardiology diagnostics
- Electron beam computerized tomography (EBCT/SPECT)
- Hysterectomy

4. Continuous Progress

Each region or employer has similar but different challenges. Progress requires continued diligence and improvement over time. High-value TPAs recommend and implement solutions to further this goal—the work is never done.

5. Positive Financial Outcomes

Depending on the size and location of the employer, employee demographics, strategies implemented, and regional health care dynamics, financial outcomes may be immediate or unfold over time. For example, an employer investing in direct primary care may see increased costs in the first year as employees begin to work through delayed health issues and adopt healthier behaviors. Often, these costs are recouped several times over in years two and three. It is also important to understand which costs can be influenced and which cannot. A high-value, transparent TPA may deliver tangible savings in utilization or unit costs even if you have an overall increase in health care expenditures due to a greater than expected number of high-cost events.

6. Engaged, Satisfied Employees

Saving money in health care requires employees to be educated, engaged participants in their health. Not all employees welcome this responsibility. However, the best TPAs build trust and empower individuals through education and reinforcement of good choices. Overall, they help save money and please employees at the same time.

How Can You Ensure Quality?

It may feel like you're venturing into foreign territory. You're not the first to act to get your employees and you a better deal, so reach out to those who have already benefited from using a high-value TPA, starting with other employers in your area. Here are two resources to help you navigate the path.

Business Groups on Health are nonprofit organizations that support employers in purchasing and managing health care benefits.

Catalyst for Payment Reform is an independent, national non-profit organization for employers committed to a higher-value health care system that can help navigate complex changes in value-based payment models.

What Challenges Can You Expect?

Administrative Challenges

Your broker, consultant, or benefits manager may be unable or unwilling to facilitate a true evaluation of TPA attributes (retention bonuses from ASOs being the primary reason).

Employee Education

A high-value, transparent TPA can sometimes feel like more of a change than employees are willing to undertake. Education about why you are tackling health care costs directly is critical to fostering more engaged employees.

Fear of Change

There is extraordinary inertia in health care. Most company benefits departments prefer not to rock the boat and stay with known vendors, even when those vendors don't perform.

Conflicts of Interest

Many brokers have undisclosed financial arrangements that favor the status quo and/or incentivize higher health care costs.

What Action Steps Can You Take?

Ask your broker, consultant, or local business group on health if they are currently working with or have experience with a high-value, transparent TPA.

Encourage your broker, consultant, or benefits manager to arrange presentations from TPAs operating in your market.

Revamp your RFPs and annual service provider evaluations to incorporate attributes of high-value, transparent TPAs. Ask your high-value, primary care provider which TPAs they like to work with.

Review all responses to your RFP, not just the ones with the lowest quotes. Sometimes value is not apparent from just looking at the bottom line numbers.

Additional Resources

Please go to healthrosetta.org/health-rosetta for ongoing updates, including lists of high-value, transparent TPA organizations, case studies, best practices, toolkits, and more.

CHAPTER 25

TRANSPARENT PHARMACY BENEFITS

"Sunlight is the best disinfectant." – William O. Douglas

Transparent Pharmacy Benefits should offer purchasers the ability to gain control of decision making based on factual, fully disclosed information. Before we get started though, it's worth noting that the term *transparency* is incredibly over-used in the market and not all transparency is created equal. It's critical to look behind any seemingly impressive pricing or numbers to get to the real underlying issues that drive costs. I only use the term here for lack of a better one.

Let's start with the key elements and goals of true Transparent Pharmacy Benefits (TPB).

1. It enables better decisions regarding pharmacy benefits, based on data that the purchaser rightly owns.
2. It provides identifiable and measurable metrics to enable informed pricing and operational control over Pharmacy Benefit Manager (PBM) services.
3. It ensures members have relevant information to make informed choices.

4. It ensures clinical decisions are based solely on efficacy and actual cost, thereby advancing the purchaser's best interests ahead of a vendor's best interests.

Why Should You Support It?

Supporting TPB is positive for almost all parties involved. Reducing therapy costs encourages patients to become more engaged in their therapy. When drug charges are unaffordable, patients won't fill their prescriptions. And there are literally thousands of opportunities where, with proper information and education, they can make better financial choices and even improve the chances of a quality outcome.

Tim Thomas, CEO of Crystal Clear Rx, gave the following example. Metformin, a valuable drug for treating diabetes, has been around for decades. It is a twice-a-day drug and can be obtained for less than $40 a month. Today, there are new formulations of Metformin that can be taken once a day, possibly improving patient adherence, but at a much greater cost to patient and employer at more than $3,000 a month. If patients were educated and properly incentivized, would they be able to maintain adherence to the older form of Metformin for a savings of nearly $36,000 per year? Pharmacists that have additional training and are paid appropriately for their time can help patients with this situation.

How Does It Work?

Unlike some Health Rosetta components, Transparent Pharmacy Benefits don't actually work much differently than what you're used to. The primary difference is the process of engaging your consultant or PBM services vendor, which focuses on contracts, access to data, and distribution channels for accessing drugs that counteract the pricing opacity, undisclosed financial incentives, and other conflicts that permeate status quo pharmacy benefits. The most critical piece is the role and involvement of an expert who knows the space top to bottom and has incentives aligned with your interests.

What Are the Key Elements to Look For?

1. Clarity on How PBMs Work

PBM business models and revenue streams are often highly complex and full of conflicts that make their incentives very different than your or your plan members' incentives. To start, they are often incentivized to push certain prescription brands. "Rebates" can be up to 25% of the total cost of a brand or specialty drug but rarely benefit the member as they are actually paid to the plan sponsor or health plan; in fact, their savings come at the expense of the patient through increased drug costs at the point of sale. Plus, the definition of what is a rebate payable to the plan sponsor or health plan rarely aligns with the actual amount paid by pharmaceutical manufacturers to the PBM. By obfuscating rebates, PBMs have found many employers will simply throw up their hands and give up, so the practice persists to their advantage. True transparency means one can see the relevant contracts the PBM has with manufacturers and others.

Some PBMs also employ pricing tactics that create "spread pricing," in which the amount charged to you and your members or a health plan is drastically higher than what is actually paid to the pharmacy. Spread pricing occurs across brand, specialty, and generic drugs. It's especially egregious in the generic space.

2. Access to Your Claims Data

Pharmacy claims data is some of the most robust and readily available in the health care industry, but first you need to get access to it, then fully understand and use it.

Your PBM relationship and agreements should make clear that you own your claims data as the purchaser of services. This includes your right to use that data to make informed decisions.

You should combine your data with other analytical resources to analyze the true cost of pharmacy treatments and not depend solely on information the PBM provides.

Access to this data is essential to operating an effective ERISA plan. ERISA health plan service providers typically abdicate fiduciary responsibilities in their contracts with your plan. This means not getting data can increase your own risk under ERISA's fiduciary requirements to manage the plan solely for the benefit of the plan members.

3. Complete Contract Understanding

Using a neutral third-party consultant to help you gain a complete understanding of current PBM contracts will ensure you have a clear understanding of current terms and conditions that are often the source of hidden costs. Even definitions left in *or out* of a contract can be financially devastating. Something as seemingly mundane as the definition of a generic can have a major impact on your spending.

This is especially true when it comes to "guarantees" in the PBM-purchaser contract. Average Wholesale Price (AWP), with its associated "discount," is the common method for evaluating PBM financial performance. AWP really means "Any Wild-assed Price" or, to be less snarky, "Ain't What's Paid." Because AWP is often confusing and misleading, it can reduce leverage in negotiations.

Scott Haas, an industry expert, provided Figure 12 on the next page as an example of how AWP can and often does produce pricing variability to the detriment of the plan sponsor and member. It is data from a real contract with a uniform AWP–68.5 percent discount for retail generics. First, notice that the price per unit varies dramatically, even though this is supposedly a uniform discount. Second, the unit costs rise over time. PBMs will say this is your cost trend, but it's often the PBM increasing cost basis to increase their spread (and revenue) over time. As a result, AWP-based discounts and metrics make it far harder to see or manage actual spending. Another issue is distribution channel pricing variability, such as mail order and specialty.

The foregoing are just a few examples of how the many moving pieces of PBM contracts, claims processing approaches, and business practices can make it difficult to manage spend. You need the right oversight and contract terms.

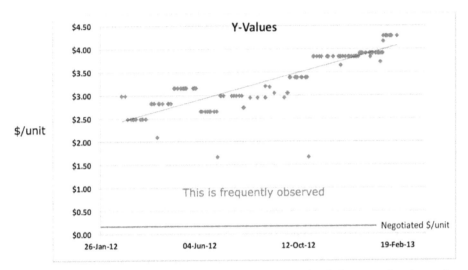

Figure 17: The contracted AWP-68.5% discount remained the same for the entire period. Each point represents a single claim. Source: Scott Haas.

4. Expert Resources

To negotiate better PBM contracts, purchasers should pair their own data with an unbiased consultant's analytical know-how, pharmacy industry knowledge, and vendor insight. Then they can decide for themselves if they should leave all of the PBM services with one vendor or if they should carve out certain aspects of the pharmacy benefit.

Consultants who only work with PBMs that pay them fees that may or may not be disclosed should be avoided. Having the wrong economic incentives makes it nearly impossible to act in the best interests of their clients. Many PBM coalitions should also be looked at with suspicion because of the lack of overall transparency and potential fiduciary duty issues under ERISA.

Follow the money before trusting any arrangement that doesn't let you view the contract between the PBM and coalition sponsor. Without it, you can't fully assess whether that arrangement will truly deliver the value represented.

5. Creative Distribution Channels

What if mail order prescriptions are actually costing you more than the same drug at retail? Seriously, this happens. When evaluating a PBM's channels, consider carving out mail order and specialty pharmacy services from the contract. Some mail order and specialty pharmacies offer services for "cost plus a management fee," which can be far less expensive than the AWP "Ain't What's Paid" model. Plan design often drives whether this is a cost-effective solution.

What Challenges Can You Expect?

1. The Appearance of Savings

Consultants and PBMs will use AWP discounts that *appear* to create significant cost savings. Remember, AWP is a flawed metric for analysis that clouds true costs and any potential savings. A good analogy for this core flaw is what happens when you multiply percentages of percentages; the math quickly gets so convoluted that it just doesn't work well.

During the RFP process, most consultants send your current pharmacy claims data to other PBMs, who then reprice the claims, showing you what you would have paid under their pricing (again, often using AWP). Since every proposal always has the appearance of savings, you'd think just doing an RFP each year would give you negative pharmacy costs eventually. Unfortunately, this isn't the case.

The core problem here is the flawed process. When your consultant just hands a potential vendor your data and has nothing to do with the repricing calculations, how can he or she have any real confidence that the work is being done correctly? Plus, very few consultants compare actual pharmacy claims to original RFP responses to ensure the original representations actually materialized in reality after the contract was signed.

A better process is for your consultant to, first, provide very basic summary information to PBM vendors about your plan, employees, total spend, prices paid through various channels, and other plan design elements; then require PBMs to provide brand and specialty pricing, plus fixed per pill unit costs for generics (usually around 3,000 of them) that include some guaranteed pricing or a Maximum Allowable Cost list; and finally, apply the responses to your actual data to create a cost-avoidance summary that shows accurate and statistically validated cost saving potential (absent specialty utilization).

This is a simplification of the process, but the key point is you need someone who applies the type of statistical discipline that would make an auditor proud. Handing data over to health plans or PBMs without provable validation controls isn't enough.

2. Interference

Many PBMs talk transparency, but it is *not* in their best financial interests. Existing consultants who are being incentivized by payments from PBMs may interfere with your journey toward transparency, as it may not be in their best financial interest.

3. Lack of Understanding

Although this may not be an obvious pain point, there still might be a lack of understanding in the HR department about the benefits of Transparent Pharmacy Benefits, or they may simply be unaware of the options available. It is important to gain HR and executive buy-in.

4. Not All Transparency Is Equal

There is often confusion between transparent and transparent pass-through. Transparent does not necessarily mean you are getting pass-through pricing and the pricing being passed through may not be the best available. Make sure you understand the different models and that the transparency is working its way to you and in your favor. Just because a vendor claims to be transparent doesn't mean they're the best option, able to secure the best pricing, or even meaningfully transparent.

5. Obfuscation to Preserve Status Quo

Consultants and PBM's who aren't forward-looking may fall back on "fear, uncertainty, and doubt" tactics meant to freeze progress. As stewards of your organization's and employees' hard-earned money, you must choose whether to protect your own health and bottom line or that of your vendor.

What Action Steps Can You Take?

Ask your broker, consultant, advisor, insurance carrier, or TPA if they are currently working with or have experience with transparent pharmacy benefits.

Ask your broker, consultant, or advisor if they or their firm receive any compensation from any PBMs or service provider?

Ask these same parties how they recognize the difference between good and bad pricing?

Encourage your broker, consultant, advisor, insurance carrier, or TPA to find, interpret, and share reliable cost and quality data from pharmacy benefits managers competing for your business.

Consider comparing pharmacy benefits managers through a structured and disciplined RFP process.

Get access to your own data to go beyond AWP and other misleading cost metrics to help you understand the real prices you're paying for each drug in your plan.

Additional Resources

Please visit healthrosetta.org/health-rosetta for ongoing updates, including lists of vendors, case studies, best practices, toolkits, and more.

CHAPTER 26

"ERISA FIDUCIARY RISK IS THE LARGEST UNDISCLOSED RISK I'VE SEEN IN MY CAREER"

Written with Sean Schantzen

The Employee Retirement Income Security Act of 1974 (ERISA) is a federal law that sets minimum standards for most voluntarily established pension and health plans in private industry to protect the individuals in these plans. Plan trustees (typically company boards, plan administrators, and others) have fiduciary duties to ERISA plans to ensure these protections are implemented and managed.

Most people know the law in relation to retirement benefits, but it is emerging as an unexpected, yet high-potential, opportunity to drive change in the dysfunctional U.S. health care system. This is because roughly 100 million Americans receive health benefits through self-insured ERISA plans, accounting for more than $1 trillion in annual health care spending (including out-of-pocket spending by plan members). Companies spend roughly double on ERISA health plans what they spend on ERISA retirement plans.

Increased outside scrutiny of how ERISA-regulated health plans spend their dollars is creating immense potential liability for companies, officers, directors, and even health insurers across the country. We are also starting to see this in benefits departments—one entire benefits department at a large, well-known company was fired (with the exception of one person) when their board became aware of the lack of proper management.

While employer and union health plans are roughly one-half of all health care spending, they likely represent over two-thirds of health care industry profits because they often wildly overpay for health care services.

This is also where a large opportunity to reduce legal risk and increase financial performance exists. Health care is the last major bucket of operating expenses that most companies still aren't actively optimizing and managing like similarly large P&L line items. This makes ERISA plans an attractive target for operational efficiencies.

Doing this is simpler than most think. ERISA requires plan trustees to prudently manage health plan assets. Yet very few health plans have the functional equivalent of an ERISA retirement plan administrator who actively manages and drives effective allocation of plan investments, either internally or externally. This person or team should have the deep actuarial and health care expertise highlighted at the end of Chapter 11, something traditional human resource departments usually lack.

Employers can also do something about the enormous fraud and waste in the system. As we saw in Chapter 8, most employers are doing little or nothing to prevent fraud because they typically aren't aware of its extent or that it's even happening. *The Economist* has reported that fraudulent health care claims alone consume $272 billion of spending each year across both private plans and public programs like Medicare and Medicaid.[176] The Institute of Medicine's study on waste in the U.S. health care system concluded that $750 billion, or 25% of all spending, is waste.[177] It's impossible to imagine any CEO, CFO, or board allowing this in any other area of their company.

Could Emerging Litigation Be Our Savior?

Key events suggest that increased scrutiny of ERISA fiduciary duties is upon us.

First, two Big Four accounting firms have refused in certain circumstances to sign off on audits that don't make allowances for ERISA fiduciary risk. At a meeting Dave attended in the last year, a senior risk management practice leader at one of those firms told a room of health care entrepreneurs and experts that ERISA fiduciary risk was the largest undisclosed risk they'd seen in their career. As more accounting firms follow suit, it could require employers to change how they manage ERISA health plans.

Second, independent board directors have quietly sounded the alarm to auditors of three separate companies (that I'm aware of) about the potential for personal financial liability that director and officer insurance policies may not cover. We expect to see more focus on this issue, given that health care spending is roughly 20 percent of payroll spending for most companies.

Third, regulatory scrutiny is beginning to increase on a number of fronts. Here's just one example. In September 2017, the Department of Labor brought a case against Macy's and two of its third-party administrators alleging violations of ERISA's fiduciary rules, largely relating to payment of out-of-network health care claims.[178] It also included alleged violations of some newer wellness program rules. This is just one example of various types of attention and scrutiny we see emerging.

Fourth, attorneys are actively cultivating cases and litigation strategies in which employers will file suits against their ERISA plan co-trustees or vendors, primarily the plan administrators who actively manage the plan's health dollars. These strategies center on allegations that the co-trustees or vendors breached ERISA fiduciary duties or other related duties by turning a blind eye to fraudulent claims. We expect the number of these cases to significantly increase in the next few years. One firm we're aware of is cultivating dozens.

The implications of this fourth trend could be enormous: If boards and plan trustees know meaningful fraud could exist and don't act to rectify the issues, they could open themselves to liability from shareholders, plan beneficiaries, and others. The magnitude of damages just for fraudulent claims could be similar to those in asbestos and tobacco lawsuits. Conservative fraudulent claims estimates are about five percent and many believe 10-15 percent is more accurate.[179] Employers spend more than $1 trillion per year through ERISA health benefits plans. Extrapolating the five percent estimate over ERISA's six-year lookback period for damages from fiduciary duty breaches, this could create $300 billion in potential damages.

These potentially significant legal risks should prompt employers to more actively manage health spending the same way they manage other large operating expenses. As we've seen, companies already doing this are reducing their health benefits spending by 20 percent or more while providing superior benefits packages.

They use a variety of approaches, but most are relatively straightforward and focus on proven benefits-design solutions that make poor care decisions more costly and better care decisions less costly. Most importantly, they don't focus on shifting costs to employees, but on tackling pricing failure, fraud, overuse, misdiagnosis, and sub-optimal treatment—the sources of most wasted spending. Finally, there are people who can help companies of all sizes implement these solutions and build better-managed plans.

Repeatedly, we've found that the best way to slash costs is to improve health benefits.

ERISA Sample Plan Document Checklist

The Department of Labor describes the fiduciary duty and potential liability as follows:

Fiduciaries have important responsibilities and are subject to standards of conduct because they act on behalf of participants in a group health plan and their beneficiaries. These responsibilities include:

- Acting solely in the interest of plan participants and their beneficiaries and with the exclusive purpose of providing benefits to them;
- Carrying out their duties prudently;
- Following the plan documents (unless inconsistent with ERISA);
- Holding plan assets (if the plan has any) in trust; and
- Paying only reasonable plan expenses.

Liability

With these fiduciary responsibilities, there is also potential liability. Fiduciaries who do not follow the basic standards of conduct may be personally liable to restore any losses to the plan, or to restore any profits made through improper use of the plan's assets resulting from their actions.

If an employer contracts with a plan administrator to manage the plan, the employer is responsible for the selection of the service provider, but is not liable for the individual decisions of that provider. However, an employer is required to monitor the service provider periodically to assure that it is handling the plan's administration prudently. To keep from falling short, fiduciaries should address the following items of language in negotiations with vendors and/or providers. (These are general guidelines to use as a starting point; please consult your own ERISA attorney for specific advice and a more comprehensive assessment.)

Allowable Payment Amounts

- "Usual and customary" or similar language is by far the most common way that health plans cut costs. Definitions of this term vary from very weak to very strong. Ideal language allows the plan administrator to pay the lesser of certain amounts based on costs, Medicare allowable amounts, etc., although a negotiated rate should always be paid to avoid breaching a network or direct contract.
- Although any claim can potentially be negotiated with the right tools, this is much more difficult if the plan document does not have language permitting negotiation (and falling back to low "usual and customary rates" in the absence of a negotiation).
- Wrap networks accessed by plans can result in little cost-savings with high fees. For this reason, we recommend an unwrapped service, which helps the plan define a reasonable and fair market, value-based allowable amount for all out-of-network claims – including those that would otherwise be sent to wrap networks – with defensible claims repricing, patient advocacy, and back-end balance-billing support to boot.

Experimental or Investigational

- "Experimental" should explicitly reference criteria such as industry-standards, accepted medical practice, service rendered on a research basis, clinical trials, and peer-reviewed literature.
- Noteworthy facets of this language that are sometimes brought into question include off-label drugs and compound drugs. The plan should clearly state how it will treat such claims.

Medical Necessity

As long as it defines medical necessity based on objective criteria, this language should be acceptable. Ideal criteria include treatment meant to restore health and otherwise appropriate under the circumstances according to the AMA or other sources. It does not include treatment that is maintenance or custodial in nature or disallowed by Medicare.

Make sure the language does not leave the determination of medical necessity to the discretion of the treating provider; the plan administrator should always retain this discretion.

Plan Administrator Discretion

- While every plan document necessarily gives the plan administrator discretion to determine payment amounts, watch out for instances where the administrator has too much or not enough discretion. Discretion should be granted to interpret the plan document's provisions and determine issues of fact related to claims for benefits.
- A provision to cover nearly anything the administrator deems appropriate may well cause a stop-loss reimbursement issue.

Fiduciary Duties

- For both self-funding veterans and those new to the industry, managing the fiduciary duties associated with making claims determinations can be a daunting task.
- Outsourcing fiduciary duties for final-level internal appeals is the most efficient and cost-effective way of handling this responsibility. Leading ERISA firms provide an approach that shifts the fiduciary burden of handling final-level appeals onto a neutral third party.

Coordination of Benefits

- If the plan is always the primary payer, that presents a cost-containment problem; It should pay secondary in all conceivable situations (except for Medicare or when otherwise not permitted) and clearly say so in the plan document.
- Ideal language will describe which plan pays primary/secondary in certain circumstances.

Leaves of Absence

- Many health plans provide coverage for any period of approved leave as determined by the employer. This can translate into individuals being covered based solely on "internal" leave policies of the employer, which are sometimes not even written, or determined on a case-by-case basis by the employer.
- While this is not a problem for the plan document per se, it is a very common problem when it comes to stop-loss reimbursement for claims incurred while an employee is on such an approved leave of absence.

Employee Skin in the Game

- Some employers elect to offer members certain incentives for performing tasks such as choosing certain providers over others, auditing bills for correctness, and purchasing durable medical equipment online at discounted rates rather than from hospitals.
- Typical rewards include offering the member a percentage of savings achieved by the plan or waiving coinsurance and deductibles.

Exclusions

- The plan document should exclude claims that result from "illegal acts." There are different ways to structure this exclusion that can increase or decrease the potential for exposure.

- Another important exclusion is for claims resulting from "hazardous activities," i.e., activities with a greater-than-normal likelihood of injury.

Overpayment Recovery and Third-Party Recovery

- To maximize recoveries, the plan document needs both strong language describing the plan's reimbursement rights and a partnership with a recovery vendor that excels at enforcing the plan's rights.
- Third-party recovery provisions should include:
- Disclaimer of the "made-whole" and "common fund" doctrines.
- Ability to recover from estates, wrongful death proceeds, and the legal guardians of minors.
- Ability to offset any funds recovered by the patient but unpaid to the plan.

Compliance and General Drafting

- The terms of the plan document must be compliant with applicable law, including ERISA, HIPAA, COBRA, and many others, in addition to any applicable state law.

Sean Schantzen was previously a securities attorney involved in representing boards, directors, officers, and companies in securities litigation, corporate transaction, and other matters. He is my co-founder in the Health Rosetta.

Please visit healthrosetta.org/health-rosetta for ongoing updates, including lists of vendors, case studies, best practices, toolkits, and more.

CONCLUSION

I often think about a question that should make us all step back a bit. Why are millennials—the largest American generation in history and largest portion of today's workforce—the first generation to think life won't be better for them than their parents?[180] In a nation of optimists, this is worrisome at best. I've come to realize that the cost of health care is a primary underlying cause: over half of their lifetime earnings are on track to go to health care and their contemporaries are dying of opioid and benzos overdoses at extraordinary rates.[181]

As millennials have children and their sense of indestructibility fades, they are realizing that they're going to be indentured servants to the health care system if it isn't broadly transformed. This is profoundly sobering, but the good news is we've solved tougher problems and this one has already been solved in microcosms around the country. The opioid crisis—seeing family members and friends dying of an entirely avoidable cause inflicted by an out-of-control health care system—gives people who wouldn't otherwise have had the resolve to tackle these issues immense energy.

There is every reason for hope. Using the simple, practical, proven fixes you've read about here, health care is getting fixed community by community. This has been the historic pattern for many of society's biggest challenges such as the Shop Local movement revitalizing local economies.

Smart benefits programs make wise decisions free or near-free and bad decisions expensive. At root, it's this simple. So-called experts who suggest the situation is too complicated to solve are often so mired in today's wildly underperforming status quo that they can't see the simple solutions hidden in plain view. Plus, status quo protectors are quite adept at making health care *seem* far more complex than necessary.

As Dan Munro likes to say, "the [health care] system was never broken, it was designed this way."[182] The best way to describe the status quo payment system is a Gordian Knot designed by Rube Goldberg. Brain surgery *is* complex. Cancer *is* complex. Building a high performing health benefits plan doesn't need to be.

Perhaps the most common corporate platitude is "our employees are our greatest asset." If that's the case, current health benefits aren't exactly delivering a great ROI. Wise leaders have realized that they operate a health care business, whether they like it or not. They also realize it's the last major budget line item they haven't optimized or brought into the modern world. Over the last 20 years, employers have increased total employee payroll spending dramatically, yet most of us don't see the benefits because it has largely gone to health care benefits costs. Forward-looking employers are putting more money in their employees' pockets while delivering superior care, driving significant financial improvements, and creating a higher performance workforce

If it wasn't already clear, true fixes to our health care mess aren't coming from D.C. The latest attempts at "reform" by Congress are yet another example of rearranging deckchairs on the Titanic: Doubling down on paying into a "system" that has no correlation between price and value and that sees 10,000 incidents of serious harm and hundreds of deaths from preventable medical mistakes every day is the definition of insanity.[183]

Hundreds of thousands of community leaders, regular citizens, clinicians, union leaders, and others are restoring the American Dream one community and organization at a time. They're stepping up in grass-roots groups and working together to solve the crisis. They're rallying around Health 3.0, the Health Rosetta,

Shatterproof, the Right Care Alliance, Stop the Addiction Fatality Epidemic (S.A.F.E.), the We the Patients movement, and many more. This is what America does. When it comes to big societal problems like civil rights, better food, or energy independence—we're best at solving these problems from the bottom up.

My purpose in writing this book and in creating the Health Rosetta was to make it simple for you to recreate these successes in your own community and across America. Now that you have the tools, you can get started today.

5 Simple Steps to Start Implementing High-Performance Benefits

The Health Rosetta was created to certify the people, products, services, and places that simplify adoption of successful approaches. We'll help you get started at healthrosetta.org. First, a few reminders:

- As much as half of health care spending provides no value. Imagine allowing any other budget line item to perform this poorly. It's unimaginable.
- Technology, vendors, and service providers that can help remove this wasteful spending while improving your employees' health already exist. They can drive far better outcomes and lower costs than status quo health plans.
- Favoring high performance vendors and services providers is a huge win for you and your employees. It also helps solve our country's health care crisis.

With this in mind, here are 5 specific next steps you can and should take.

Reset your benefits advisor relationship expectations.

Employers deeply rely on a benefits advisor, consultant, or broker to navigate this complex world. In our experience, less than five percent of benefits brokers and consultants are worthy of that trust. They have deep expertise and tremendous commitment to their clients' best interests. A litmus test for whether yours falls into this group is to ask them to complete and sign the compensation disclosure form in Appendix D. The high performers will have no problem agreeing to this long before you make any benefits purchasing decisions. If they hesitate, make excuses, or refuse, that should be a deal-breaker. I'd encourage you to find a high-performance benefits advisor or consultant by following the guidance in Chapter 12.* You need someone on your side.

In tandem, evaluate the plan administrator you are working with. Chapters 15 and 24 address the shortcomings and conflicts-of-interest of many plan administrators and what you should expect from an optimal plan administrator.

Start now and select approaches that minimize disruption to your benefits group.

Don't be a slave to the annual benefits process. It's largely designed for a broker's or health plan's convenience, not your objectives. Many high-performance strategies can be implemented any time of the year. It often makes sense to do this off-cycle to manage your benefits group's workload. Solutions to reverse the opioid crisis continue to emerge and come throughout the year – waiting costs lives.

Build compounding momentum by implementing programs that quickly reduce spending and deliver value.

Part IV of the book (Chapters 21-26) summarizes a few of the Health Rosetta's highest impact components, proven to deliver

---

* *Healthrosetta.org/employers has more resources, including a calculator to show the EBITDA impact of high-performance health benefits and the revenue you'd need to generate to create similar impact.*

* *The Health Rosetta certifies transparent, mission-aligned benefits advisors and others. Naturally, there are great advisors who aren't yet aware of this certification, so you might have one that isn't yet certified. However, the Health Rosetta is doing the utmost to identify, accept, and hold accountable as many of the strongest performers as possible.*

improved health outcomes and drive significant savings in relatively short order, usually within 12 months. They quickly free resources by addressing big ticket items like pricing failures, fraud, overtreatment, misdiagnosis, and drug spend.

Build support by positioning these programs to employees as new, better benefits, even if they are layered on top of your current plan design. Three simple examples that work for nearly any size organization and don't require geographically concentrated workforces are pharmacy analysis/optimization, Centers of Excellence models, and out-of-network claims settlement services. I also recommend using some of the initial savings to fund further programs, as this compounds momentum.

You'll likely need help from a high-performance benefits advisor, but the Health Rosetta can also help navigate this process. We'll even help find an advisor willing and able to drive the process.

Develop an outstanding communications strategy to ensure program success.

Companies typically fully transition their workforce to high-performance benefits over a couple of years, creating compounding momentum each year. This requires strong employee communication.

A natural place to start is with new employees and millennials. For example, you can default new employees into new, higher value benefits programs positioned as "Tier 1." You keep the old programs as "Tier 2." (See the case study on Enovation Controls on page 238 to see how they did it.) Word will spread and people will naturally transition to Tier 1.

Millennials are often the early adopters of what everyone ultimately adopts. Health care's status quo is nearly a perfect polar opposite to what millennials want and value (e.g., convenience, transparency, etc.). See Chapter 6 on how to leverage millennials to transform your benefits. Millennials have been particularly impacted by the opioid crisis, giving them yet another driver for health benefits changes. In 2010, just 18 out of every 100,000 Americans aged 25-34 died from a drug overdose. By 2014, that rate rose to about 23 in 100,000—then it really took off. From 2014 to 2016 it spiked by 50 percent to almost 35 in 100,000. [184]

Connecting benefits changes with the desire to reverse the opioid crisis is a great way to explains the rationale for many of these changes.

Larger employers can also start phasing in changes in individual locations to work out kinks and ensure value is being delivered.

Let the Health Rosetta help guide the way.

Health Rosetta can give you access to resources, insight, and people to help navigate the process. Your path and focus will vary significantly based on your organization type, size, geography, employee base, current plan, and more. We'll help you get the lay of the land, serving as a backstop against common myths and misinformation about what you can achieve.

Restore the American Dream for Your Community

It became clear to me that I needed to write this book after seeing dozens of organizations—from small manufacturers to large municipalities to Fortune 100 companies—that have reduced their spending by 20 percent or more *while* saving their employees from avoidable harm such as opioid use disorders and financial insolvency. They spend $2,000 to $5,000 less per member every year—money that can go into employees' pockets and thus into the community. These same results are possible for nearly any purchaser that has the will and access to the right expertise. It's how you can personally help restore the American Dream.

If every employer adopts these common sense steps, we'll create a $500 billion citizen-driven economic stimulus every year while dramatically improving the lives of countless citizens.

Let's be clear about the stakes. Data from Rand, Brookings, Kaiser, Health Affairs, and other reputable sources have shown that hyperinflating health care costs have been 95 percent responsible for 20 years of income stagnation and decline for the middle class and our most vulnerable citizens. This has profoundly and negatively impacted nearly every single American. Unlike other great public health crises such as polio, the opioid crisis is entirely caused by a dysfunctional health care system. It's a national shame that we can reverse.

No industry spends anywhere near what health care does on marketing and lobbying at the local, state and federal levels. Each of us must inoculate ourselves against status quo enablers who benefit—at the cost of our health and our wealth—when they infect us with the sense that health care is too complex to fix. This is simply false and the Health Rosetta shows how and why.

Americans are no longer waiting for solutions from somewhere else. We're looking in the mirror and realizing it's on us to restore the American Dream. As you saw in this book, the fixes even transcend the lines that divide us. Remember, in Pittsburgh unions and management put aside old battles and rethought how to deliver great benefits to teachers. As a result, Pittsburgh kindergartners will have $2 billion more for education during their K-12 years than their counterparts in Philadelphia. Pittsburgh's teachers are also paid more, have better benefits, and have 30% smaller classes sizes.

Successes are being created by people across the political spectrum. Progressives are implementing approaches that some would call conservative. Conservatives are implementing approaches that some would call progressive. The common thread in each is that the people involved shifted their mindset, realizing that we don't need left-or-right, management-or-labor solutions. We need an American solution and the good news is it's spreading like wildfire.

No matter who you are, there's a way to take action.

- **Employees.** Share with your CEO, CFO, and benefits leader that they can slash health care costs while improving benefits.
- **Executives and public sector leaders.** Ignore so-called experts and apply the same discipline to purchasing health care as to every other area of your organization.

- **Union leaders.** Rethink your relationship with management in regard to the health benefits costs that have been crushing your members. When it comes to health care, you're on the same side.
- **Clinicians and health care professionals.** Buck the status quo by embracing the Health 3.0 Vision and Health Rosetta Principles outlined in Appendices D to F. We'll even help. If your organization won't do it, go to an organization that will.
- **All citizens.** Persuade those in your community to take action by telling them about the Health Rosetta or giving them this book.

No country has smarter or more compassionate nurses and doctors. No country has more innovators that have reinvented medical science time and again. Nearly every individual in health care went into it for all the right reasons, but perverse incentives and outdated approaches have left them shackled or downtrodden. Whether we knew it or not, we all contributed to this mess. Now, it's on all of us to fix it. When change happens community by community, it's impossible to stop.

Yes, health care stole the American Dream. But it's absolutely possible to take it back. Join us to make it happen in your community.

Please share a free version of this book

That's right. If you think some or all of this book is worth sharing, we created a page where our friends can share a free download of the book. We care much more about solving the problems outlined in this book than losing a few book sales. Simply send your friends and colleagues to http://www.healthrosetta.org/wakeup-call. And they can download the book for free. In fact, you should sign up there too. I regularly update the book and if you sign up, you'll receive notifications of new chapters and updated information.

ACKNOWLEDGMENTS & AUTHOR'S NOTE

Stop! Don't Skip This!

We all skip the acknowledgments, but I encourage you to read or skim for two reasons:

1. This book wouldn't be possible without insight from the pioneering individuals here and throughout the book.
2. What you've been told about fixing health care just isn't true. It's already happening from the ground up. Any benefits purchaser can follow, no matter what excuse you hear from the status quo protectors. Each of the more than 100 individuals and organizations in this book is doing it every day and each knows many others doing the same. Following the people below and the suggestions in this book can lead the way.

First, I want to acknowledge the employers, unions, their stellar benefits advisors, and others such as physician leaders who have provided the substance for this book. I highlight five employers and unions, but visit healthrosetta.org /learn/ case-studies/ for many other case studies. The common thread is that these regular citizens are problem solvers who ignore the partisan and status quo orthodoxies. They care more about enabling the American Dream.

Self-described progressives have implemented programs that many would call conservative and self-described conservatives have implemented programs that many would call progressive. Seeing this has been a breath of fresh air from the partisan bickering that dominates the health care reform conversation.

Not long ago, I knew next to nothing about health benefits. I just wanted to find (and fix) the root cause of our wildly under-performing health care system. How could we have so many smart and passionate doctors, nurses, clinicians of all types, and other professionals—and spend far more than other countries—yet have largely abysmal health outcomes? The root cause I found is that we purchase health care incredibly ineffectively. Medicare, Medicaid, private & public employers. Everywhere. I decided to focus on employers and unions for practical reasons.

1. The overwhelming majority of non-poor, non-elderly get their benefits through their job. There's no real evidence of this changing anytime soon.
2. The overwhelming majority of individuals enslaved by opioid use disorders are working age or their dependents. Further, many Medicaid recipients contending with addiction started their journey while employed. Addiction often led to losing their job and eventually becoming a Medicaid recipient.
3. As a general rule, employers and unions—including public sector employers—are especially ineffective at purchasing high value health benefits.
4. Wise public employers and unions are already showing how to dramatically increase health care investment value. This simplifies spreading the best solutions to public programs like Medicaid and Medicare.
5. Employers and unions can innovate independently without an Act of Congress or top-down master plan. The best solutions can be broadly replicated, creating a self-reinforcing dynamic to get us out of this mess.

The people below have both realized this and work tirelessly to fix our health care system from the ground up. I want to high-light just a few of the people driving this grassroots movement that have most inspired me.

Benefits Experts

Forward-leaning benefits experts are the vanguard that is worth its weight in gold. They've left behind wasteful, obsolete approaches that plague most employers. They're the architects and first members of the Health Rosetta. I can't thank them enough. They take what Margaret Mead once said to heart.

Never doubt that a small group of thoughtful, committed citizens can change the world; indeed, it's the only thing that ever has.

They've taught me virtually everything I've learned about health benefits:

Ashley Bacot, David Balinski, Jeff Bernhard, David Contorno, Heidi Cottle, Tom Emerick, Fred Goldstein, Scott Haas, Brian Klepper, Eric Krieg, Craig Lack, Lee Lewis, Jim Millaway, Andy Neary, Ron Peck, Keith Robertson, Adam Russo, Bill Rusteberg, Edward Smith, and Woody Waters.

I also want to acknowledge the first group of forward-leaning benefits advisors that we've accepted into the Health Rosetta Benefits Certification Programs:

Robson Baker, Gary Becker, Adam Berkowitz, Bret Brummitt, Josh Butler, Thomas Carey, Curtis Colbert, David Contorno, Megan Cook, Dan Cronin, Dan DaCosta, Alex Dampf, Chris Davis, Joseph Deacon, Thomas DiLiegro, Tim Doherty, Eric Dreyfus, Lori Fearon, Brian Flowerday, Mark Gall, Cary Goss, Cristy Gupton, John Harvey, Bryce Heinbaugh, Chris Hamilton, John Humkey, Chad Jackovich, Joshua Jeffries, Adam Karalius, Mark Krogulski, Justin Leader, Lee Lewis, Taylor Lindsey, Donnie Marcontell, Tracy McConnell, Keith McNeil, Matt McQuide, Jared Meays, Jim Millaway, Kalli Ortega, Ashley Pace, Mike Patton, Rebeccah Randles, Dan Ross, Robert Sankey, John Sbrocco, Carl Schuessler, Jr., Darrell Schwabe, Craig Scurato, Richard Silberstein, Bradley Smith, Edward Smith, Thomas Stautberg, Tommy Taylor, Antione

Turner, Brian Uhlig, Chris Van Buren, Mark Weber, Rex Wilcox, and Tina Wilt.

Delivery System Innovators

These individuals give me hope. They're just a sampling of those I've been honored to learn from. The common thread is they're believers and doers on my favorite quote by Buckminster Fuller:

"You never change things by fighting the existing reality. To change something, build a new model that makes the existing model obsolete."

The path to success is bumpy. Each of these individuals has faced many setbacks and keeps bouncing back:

Drs. Erika & Garrison Bliss, Jeff Butler, Dr. Natasha Burgert, Dr. Christopher Crow, Dr. Rushika Fernandopulle, Jon Hernandez, Dr. Howard Luks, Dr. Sachin Jain, Dr. Marty Makary, Dr. Andrey Ostrovsky, Dr. Jay Parkinson, Dr. Jerry Reeves, Mason Reiner, Ryan Schmid, Dr. Jordan Shlain, Dr. Prabhjot Singh, Dr. Michael Sprintz, Dr. Wendy Sue Swanson, Dr. Craig Tanio, Dr. Bill Thomas, Dr. Bryan Vartabedian, Dr. Sue Woods, Dr. Sheldon Zinberg, and the late Dr. Tom Ferguson.

The Health Innovation Ecosystem

I greatly appreciate the individuals who have invited me to their events and podcasts that advance my thinking and help spread this book's message of hope:

Steve Ambrose, Tom Banning, Jessica Brooks, Mike Ferguson, Nelson Griswold, Gautam Gulati, Fard Johnmar, Vidar Jorgensen, Laurel Pickering, Stacey Richter, Kevin Trokey and Karen van Caulil.

Other health innovators have greatly helped shape my thinking for the book:

Mark Blum, Chris Brookfield, Shannon Brownlee, Jonathan Bush, Dave deBronkart, Esther Dyson, Dr. Vivek Garipalli, Mark Gaunya, Dr. Venu Julapalli, Dr. Vinay Julapalli, Leonard Kish, Jan Oldenburg, Marc Pierson, Josh Luke, Kat Quinn, Dr. Vikas Saini, Bassam Saliba, Dr. Danny Sands, Dr. Martin Sepulveda, Chris Shoffner, Holly Spring, Melissa Taylor, and Tim Thomas.

Inspirational Authors

I'd also like to thank the authors of some great books that shaped my thinking:

Tom Emerick & Al Lewis (Cracking Health Costs), Deborah & James Fallows (Our Towns), Dr. Atul Gawande (Being Mortal), David Goldhill (Catastrophic Care), Dr. Marty Makary (Unaccountable), Dr. Robert Pearl (Mistreated), Sam Quinones (Dreamland), Cathryn Jakobson Ramin (Crooked), Elisabeth Rosenthal (An American Sickness), Paul Shoemaker (Can't Not Do), Nassim Taleb (Antifragile), John Torinus (The Company that Solved Healthcare), and many others.

I'm thankful for those I follow on Twitter—twitter.com/chasedave/ following. I constantly weed and feed that list with a self-imposed 100 follow limit. This makes it my most useful tool for keeping up with the industry.

The Book Team

Lauren Phillips led the book's editing effort. Her depth in health care didn't hamper her ability to make the book readable for people outside of health care. She was a delight to work with.

I also want to specially thank my partner in the Health Rosetta, Sean Schantzen. Without him, there's no way I could advance the Health Rosetta ecosystem like we are. He's an unofficial editor and has added critical depth to the book, uses his legal background to keep me out of hot water, oversees our investing, launched the Health Rosetta certification program, and has been key to executing our strategy to grow the Health Rosetta ecosystem. Perhaps most importantly, he's fundamentally driven by a similar mission as I am. Scaling broad adoption of simple, proven, non-partisan fixes to our health care system has become the thing he can't not do.

Rounding out our team are Ellyn Howard, Robin Schantzen and Melissa Taylor. They all contributed to myriad different facets of putting the book together and getting it in your hands.

The Fuel to My Fire

I wouldn't be fully candid if I didn't mention the nearly daily fuel I receive from the stories of organizations and individuals acting with impunity to protect their interests at great expense to society. Here are just two examples.

1. Executives at one of the largest tax-exempt, faith-based hospitals systems in the country threatening electoral retaliation against the mayor of a city. Why? The mayor wanted to provide far better primary care to employees than the hospital system was providing. This would have allowed the city to balance its budget and provide better services to citizens.

2. An executive at one of the largest insurance companies in the country knowingly turning a blind eye to literally billions of dollars of fraud (see Chapter 9 for details) being perpetrated against the employees and employers they process claims for. One of the impacted companies (a heartland manufacturer) laid off 10,000 workers—many of which could have been saved if not for the $100s of millions of clearly fraudulent claims paid by the company.

The Best Part of My Life

Last, but certainly not least—my family. Almost everything I write goes past Coleen for review. If something I write isn't comprehensible, it's usually because I didn't run it by her. Our kids, Abby & Cam, warn people to not bring up health care with me unless they have hours of available discussion time. I'm, by far, the worst writer of the family. I look forward to reading their work in the future.

They have heard more about health care than anyone should have to, yet still have the sense of humor to give me grief about it. They may not know it, but a core reason I'm maniacal about building a much-improved health ecosystem is that I want to do my part to leave them with a much better health ecosystem than when I arrived. God has blessed me with a great family and great kids. I'm on a mission to ensure everyone has the same opportunities for full health that we have.

APPENDIX A

EVIDENCE-BASED SERVICES FOR PEOPLE WITH OPIOID USE DISORDER*

Type of Service	Nature and Purpose	Advantages	Concerns
Detoxification/ Stabilization	· Generally provided in hospital · Manages acute crisis safely · Removes opioids from body if needed prior to treatment	· Reduces immediate medical risk · Gives opportunity to engage patient in treatment	· Without follow-up treatment, patient at higher risk of overdose due to loss of tolerance
Opioid Agonist Therapy	· Outpatient care in specialty clinic (methadone) or primary care (buprenorphine) · Transitions patient away from more dangerous opioids (e.g., heroin) and use routes (e.g., injection)	· Extremely strong clinical trial evidence of reducing illicit drug use, infectious disease transmission, mortality, and crime · Provides biological stabilization that allows patients to engage in employment or vocational training/ counseling	· Methadone and buprenorphine are opioids with street value and may be diverted for sale/ misuse · Some patients may increase alcohol consumption or other non-opioid drug use · Usually requires additional psychosocial services to be maximally effective

12-Step Facilitation Counseling	· Introduces patients to 12-step concepts · Links patients to 12-step fellowships	· Evidence of reducing all forms of drug use · Takes advantage of long-term, cost-free support for recovery (e.g. Narcotics Anonymous)	· Less effective as a standalone than when combined with medication · Some 12-step group members object to medication-assisted treatment
Therapeutic Communities	· Residential communities designed to promote abstinence and eliminate antisocial attitudes/ behaviors · Make extensive use of peer counseling · Often connected to correctional facilities	· Some evidence of reducing substance use and recidivism · May ease transition back to society for addicted prisoners	· Costly and requires long-term absence from any work and family roles · In-prison therapeutic communities without post-prison services may confer little or no benefit
Needle/Syringe Exchange	· Provides sterile injection equipment and education on reducing infectious disease risk	· Evidence of reducing HIV/AIDS transmission · May serve as a gateway to other needed services, including addiction treatment	· Probably has no effect on hepatitis C infection · Siting programs can be challenging due to community resistance · Not relevant for those who only consume opioids without injection

| Naloxone | · Antagonist medication that rapidly reverses opioid overdose

· Increasingly carried by emergency medical technicians, police officers, fire fighters, homeless shelter workers

· Sometimes distributed to drug users and their loved ones | · Low-risk medication that can be safely employed after minimal training

· Initial evidence of reducing community overdose rates

· Generic formulation is inexpensive | · Does not affect underlying addiction

· Without treatment linkage, may simply set stage for next overdose

· Can be overpowered by potent fentanyl |

STATUS QUO BENEFITS VS. HEALTH ROSETTA TYPE BENEFITS

Given the massive amount of money spent by employers on health benefits, it's brutal to look at just how bad the status quo is for health benefits. As you review Open Enrollment information, consider that roughly $10,000 is extracted from take-home pay. By comparison, wise employers are spending $5,000-$7,000 per capita with these superior benefits. Reconsider whether you are okay with the status quo. This is even more important, as most employers are going to high-deductible plans and thus what comes out of an employee's paycheck covers less and less. This make health care and health plans one of the few industries where the value proposition gets worse every year. No industry has lower Net Promoter Scores (a measure of customer satisfaction) than Health Plans. Tweaks on the margins won't get the job done.

Status Quo Versus Health Rosetta Comparison

The list of items below gives you a good punch list of what to work on. They are ordered roughly by the level of effort and disruption to the relative payback (i.e., low effort and high ROI bubbles to the top).

Transparent Advisor Relationships

Health Benefits Status Quo	Health Rosetta
"Shops" the insurance every year. Facilitates insurance purchases one year at a time. Believes costs are dependent on the best offer of the carrier. Gives limited data on where your money is going. Provides limited ways to control underlying costs. Doesn't talk about their compensation, or worse, is solely paid on commission, i.e., the more rates increase, the more income the broker receives. Advocates cost-shifting in the form of increased deductibles and copays to lower the employer impact of premium increases. Blames costs exclusively on employee behavior and poor health.	· Creates a 3-5-year plan. · Brings transparency to where the money is going. · Talks about their compensation and is willing to tie compensation to performance. · Provides risk management to suit the needs of the business owner(s). · NEVER surprises with a "shock" renewal rate. · Returns control over your costs to you. · Bring the "benefit" of Benefits back to your business. · Makes health benefits a real attraction and retention tool. · Understands *improving* benefits is the only way to lower costs. · Provides detailed data driven analysis and actionable insight.

Active, Independent Plan Management

Health Benefits Status Quo	Health Rosetta
Many ERISA plans have "holes" that expose employers unnecessarily. Pay for high cost ASO networks.	· Fully-compliant ERISA plans that protect companies from abuse. · ERISA fiduciary oversight and review at least as strong as 401k oversight and management. · Use networks focused on high quality providers and geographic coverage.

Transparent Open Networks

Health Benefits Status Quo	Health Rosetta
Wildly variant, opaque pricing for items such as scans, surgeries, and other medical services. If there is any price/quality correlation, it's inversely correlated. Sometimes "transparency" solutions are available giving the best, bad deal while still having co-pays, deductibles, the oxymoronic "Explanation of Benefits," etc. and all the other things that make for a horrible consumer experience.	The good news is there is a solution to pricing failure, the most vexing problem health care has had. Fair, fully transparent price to employer/individual at high-quality centers that readily accept quality reporting such as Leapfrog, etc. Providers able to set a price that works for them while avoiding claims/collections hassles and accompanying receivables. No charge for individual going to these providers. No bills, etc., just a thank you note.

Value-based Primary Care

Health Benefits Status Quo	Health Rosetta
Flawed reimbursement incentives have turned primary care into "loss leaders" that are like milk in the back of the grocery store (i.e., low-margin services designed to get people to high-margin services). Short appointments due to not investing properly in primary care. Primary care shortage due to making primary care discipline unappealing. Long wait times to get in can lead to small "fires" blowing up. Medically unnecessary face-to-face appointments clog the waiting room and delay care for people who truly need face-to-face encounters. Record levels of dissatisfaction & burnout amongst PCPs.	· Can fully address over 90% of the issues people enter the health care system for within a primary care setting. · Health coaching addresses lifestyle-driven conditions. · PCP is Sherpa-like resource to help navigate treacherous terrain of complex medical conditions requiring specialty care, procedures, etc. · Same- or next-day appointments for issues not addressed via email/phone. · Extensivist (for the sickest patients) has smaller panel allowing proactive care management & coordination. · Can reduce issues 40-90% and spending 20-50%. · Quadruple Aim leading organizations. · High Net Promoter Scores.

Transparent Pharmacy Benefits

Health Benefits Status Quo	Health Rosetta
Limited or no transparency and control over Pharmacy Benefit Manager (PBM) services. Actual costs often hidden or obfuscated under AWP analysis, rebates, or pseudo-transparency. Including drugs on "preferred" tiers often based on financial, not clinical efficacy, reasons.	· Provide transparency and control over Pharmacy Benefit Manager (PBM) services. · Ensure members have relevant information to make informed choices. · Ensure clinical decisions are based solely on efficacy and ACTUAL cost. · Is a process that works on behalf of the purchaser's best interests.

Benefits Concierge Service

Health Benefits Status Quo	Health Rosetta
Employees left to navigate an extremely siloed and uncoordinated health care system receiving conflicting and often non-evidence-based recommendations.	Having resources to help you navigate the system that can draw on expertise for quality and cost including understanding benefits plans, best provider options, etc.

Major Specialties & Outlier Patients

Health Benefits Status Quo	Health Rosetta
Procedures Quality and prices vary widely. Studies find 40% of transplants are medically unnecessary. High rates of complications at community hospitals who don't do high volumes of complex procedures. **Acute diseases** Little or no evidence-based or patient-specific care or treatment protocols. Highly disjointed care with little communication between providers. No defined approach to match patients to high-quality specialist providers. No access to non-physician resources to facilitate ongoing management or support.	**Procedures** Second opinions at no charge for employee at world-class Centers of Excellence facilities (e.g., Mayo & Cleveland clinics). Unit cost often higher but lower complication rates & avoidance of unnecessary procedures drives strong ROI. Due to the infrequency of these procedures (transplants, neurological procedures, cardiac, spine, and other six-figure or more procedures), this pairs well with Transparent Medical Networks for more common procedures. **Acute diseases** Access to evidence-based and disease-specific care navigation, pathways, and treatment protocols. Highly coordinated care with defined handoffs between care providers. Simple access to high-quality providers with demonstrable strong outcomes. Non-physician care team resources facilitate ongoing management and support.

APPENDIX C

A PRACTICAL HANDBOOK FOR SYSTEMS CHANGE

Applied Through Salish|Growth^{spc} *- A Community Building Company.*
By Chris Brookfield

"Triggering a widespread economic movement towards decentralization amongst thousands of independent actors."

This handbook describes a process that I have used for 12 years to develop and produce community building companies. In that time, we've recognized a process and shown that it's replicable.

The purpose of this handbook is as an internal resource at Salish | Growth and shared with interested third parties. Salish | Growth focuses on instigating commercial resilience outside of urban cores in the Salish and Columbia Watersheds.

Our work is designed to be entirely open source, and we invite active extension of this work.

Over and over, we have seen that an interdisciplinary approach that joins human focused disciplines with analytical approaches, has triggered large-scale systems change.

Please contact Chris Brookfield (cbookfield@gmail.com) or Arlen Coily (awc468@gmail.com).

- 0. Introduction
- I. Process
- II. Scale
- III. Design
- IV. Timing

0. Introduction to the Nautilus Process

This is a process of system change.

It's nothing new to you.

It has worked for us, over and over.

It can be taught. It can be learned.

Go forward, go backwards, start where you land.

Keep moving.

Systems Change – Establishing Credibility

Unitus Equity Fund - Microcredit for poor communities in India

SKS Microcredit, Bharat (Urban Microcredit)	Microcredit, entrepreneurship, and venture capital led to replication and imitation. Serving millions of families, two of our companies list publicly and one is part of IDFC Bank, a national bank in India.
Ujjivan (Rural Microcredit)	
GVFML (Place Based Microcredit)	

- 10+ million families served
- Over 20,000 jobs created
- Accelerate poor into middle class
- $5+ billion capital crowded in
- 26% Ten Year IRR - cash
- Successful systems change

Elevar - Human centered venture capital develops and funds 20+ human services companies.

Vistaar (Lending to Informal Business)	Twenty human services companies. Grown, replicated, and imitated over and over.
Shubham (Slum Home Improvement)	
Glocal (Rural Acute Health Care)	

- Demonstrates that this process of change can be replicated across diverse services.

North American Grain

Cairnspring Mills (Safe, local, identity preserved flour)	Proof of concept for food system change.

- Demonstrates that this process can be extended to North America.

I. Process

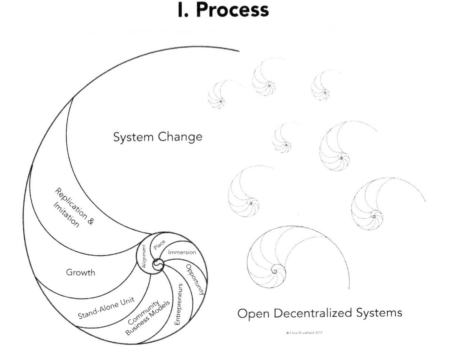

301

Alignment

Self: Identification of tension between individual/local and legacy/global systems.

Dissonance: Conflict points toward opportunities.

Synthesis: Conflicting values aligned in practice.

Resonance: Community and system values more closely aligned.

Transition: Find a place to practice.

Place

Determine scale: Small enough for local ownership, large enough for economies of scale.

Determine perimeter of focus: Constraints inspire innovative thinking.

Determine identity: Observe social, economic, and geographic organization.

Transition point: Dive into community.

Immersion

Participate: Join community.

Generate empathy: Understand community members.

Build: Personal relationships.

Perceive: Observe, listen, and receive information.

'Map': Social networks.

'Map': Market linkages.

Transition point: Identified essential community needs.

Opportunity

Connect: Needs to resources.

Identify: Barriers and bridges.

Calculate: Potential market size.

Find: Solutions that mimic existing social relationships.

***Transition point**: Effervescent community support.*

Entrepreneurs

Rooted: Deeply immersed in community.

Manage: Successful team leader.

Aligned: Active in relevant social movement.

Mindset: Clear vision, open mind.

***Transition Point**: Entrepreneur committed to system change for the benefit of their community.*

Community Business Model

Replicate: Models an effective existing relationship in the community.

Iterate: Test and replicate relationship structure.

Gauge: Acceleration of engagement (Suppliers, Clients, Capital) indicates possible model.

Community Support: Facilitates growth and removal of barriers.

***Transition**: Defined community business model.*

Stand-Alone Unit

Build: One stand-alone unit.

Book: Operational profit.

Design: Replicable financial, business, and physical model.

Transition: Successful imitation & replication.

Growth

Scale: Grow and add units.

Distribute: Encourage replication & imitation.

Raise capital: Fund expansion, new replication, and new imitation.

Transition: Business and social movement coalesce and power each other.

Replication & Imitation

Repeat: Run process again.

Open: Distribute design and process.

Support: Assist in imitation and replication.

Share: Teach and mentor process, encourage imitation.

Transition point: System changes self-propagate.

II. Scale

Watersheds

A watershed's boundaries are drawn clearly by mountains, rivers, and floodplains. At this scale, people living in a given watershed share a base of natural resources, culture, and economy. This sharing forms a basis for mutual concern. Watersheds are a natural shape for community formation. Companies may emerge at the watershed scale that reflect the needs of the underlying community. In this way, these companies share local people's pre-existing organization and needs. This partially explains why our companies have historically spent so little on marketing – we do not have to create needs, we do not have to educate consumers about our services, and we do not need to cause community structures to reorient around our distribution.

We have chosen watersheds as our default unit of scale. While we do not know whether a smaller unit, such as a neighborhood, would be better, we do know that just about the entirety of investment management is carried out on much bigger scales. Virtually all money management is national, international, or global in scale. By reducing our scale, we have found solutions and uncovered opportunities that are impossible to see from larger scales.

There appears to be an inherent validity to the watershed scale. Watersheds map very well to the human communities and economies that rest within the physical geography. When we look at these watersheds through history, we find that a great deal of the essential services were defined at this scale. Flour mills were organized by the position of rivers within watersheds. Farmers' fields and agricultural production is organized by watersheds. Towns, cities, and communities are organized by watershed. Much of our work in India was organized into catchments or watersheds.

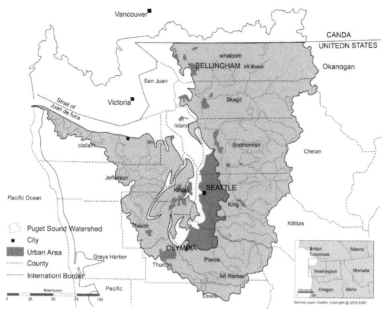

Salish Watershed

One of the insights we discovered at the watershed scale is the remarkable similarity in the network geometry in these watersheds. When the landscape is mapped at this scale, it appears to be a distributed, scale-free network branching out from the river systems. When the community - people and their relationships - are mapped to the watershed, the resultant network is very similar. Both have dense connections in the same areas, around the main stems of rivers. Both are sparse near the steep passes and uplands on the edge of the watersheds. And the amount of market activity mirrors the underlying community and physical geography. In a sense, markets as networks ride atop community and community atop the watershed. Each nested and formed with similar dimensions. Our inquiry into the Skagit River basin, where we found the flour opportunity, reflects this same organization.

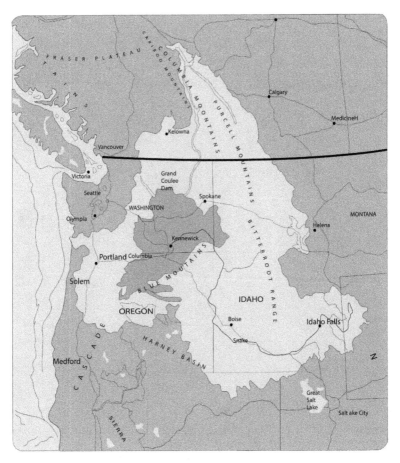

Columbia Watershed

Focus on smaller, more appropriate scales, is one aspect of how we found our flour opportunity and several of our Indian human services opportunities.

Salish | Growth is currently focused on the Salish and Columbia watersheds.

III. Design

We are particularly focused on business models that emphasize local, open, and independent attributes. When combined, these attributes create a semi-autonomous distributed network

This topology, or fabric, again reflects the same network

geometry as the underlying geography, community and commerce. The design of this business fabric echoes the designs of the nested watershed systems. In this way, the underlying systems – geography, community, and market - strengthen the business model.

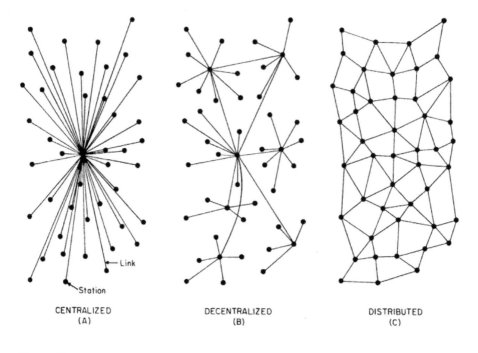

CENTRALIZED (A)

DECENTRALIZED (B)

DISTRIBUTED (C)

Local

By focusing on local, our businesses gain a number of intrinsic advantages that are often overlooked.

First, by decreasing scale, solutions can appear to problems that seem too complicated to solve at global scale. For instance, re-engineering the food system or decreasing poverty really are intractable when viewed at the global scale. Even the basic atoms of these systems, people, are invisible. By dialing into local, new features and relationships emerge. We see that poor people are economically active and can increase productivity with capital access. We see that midscale flour mills can make significant improvements to soil conservation, yields, and overall system resilience, while increasing overall consumer health and satisfaction.

Our local business models are organized in patterns of existing community organization. Our supply chains are short and use existing logistics. Our distribution uses existing networks; we are not attempting to disrupt local relationships. Our services (such as credit, insurance, health care, milling) are considered essential by the community. Because we are offering services that are NOT new, but better mapped to underlying community organization, we need very little money for marketing. We do not need to educate the customer. We do not need to induce changes in community organization. We do not have to pay for engagement. The communities we work in have already done this work for themselves through their social movements.

Open

Our business models are open. This means that we are not even attempting to take proprietary positions or defend our ideas with patents. We share our thinking and discoveries. By being open, each local implementation helps to extend the innovation. Each new watershed can adopt the change through replication and imitation.

Openness is an advantage; largely because information networks have coalesced over the past 15 years and have exponentially increased the flow of information to local communities. There is no way to transmit proprietary ideas at anywhere near the speed and coverage that open sourced ideas move. As information networks have grown, so has the relative advantage in propagating open ideas as compared to contracting proprietary property.

Other than unique names and necessarily personal aspects of our companies, the only aspect of our companies that we protect are the relationships we build. We want to protect and cherish these links to our farmers, bakers, and the community. However, where we have trust and reciprocity, we encourage sharing of relationships, as this speeds replication and imitation.

Independence

Here we mean independence of control, ownership, and production. Since each functional unit is independently owned, there is no central controller. This means that each entrepreneur controls their own brand, production methods, company culture, and resource allocations.

Because our companies are decentralized, they are free to innovate. In flour, we may end up with many variations in how each entrepreneur optimizes their business and serves their customers; choosing their own mill configurations, brands, grain varieties, and growers. By giving up our control as investors, entrepreneurs are put in position to make their own decisions, and the result is a wide diversity of approaches to similar activities. This diversity is at the heart of resilience.

The decentralized business models that are implemented across different watersheds are part of a fabric an interconnected network of autonomous entities. We are not holding proprietary control over the businesses we help start, and we do not intend to be the only ones implementing the nautilus process. We will scale the impact of this company by continuing to replicate the process in new watersheds and new verticals. We will also actively encourage imitation through openness.

As with scale, we are hybridizing our approach to system design to incorporate the best of both local and conglomerated infrastructure. By integrating business models with existing social movements, we achieve network connectivity beyond the local watershed, allowing the sharing of resources, information, and values. By allowing each of these businesses to function autonomously within this fabric and grow to their fullest individual potentials, an individual mill can utilize the control and hierarchical scalability typified by corporation. While at the same time, the fabric, as a whole, achieves quick responses, flexibility, and adaptability – responses which are inhibited by corporate concentration.

THE NATURAL WORLD IS COMPOSED OF DISTRIBUTED ARCHITECTURE

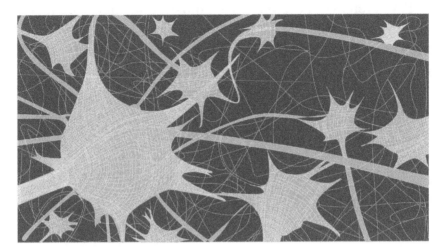

Independent Agents in a Fabric Linked Through Communication

IV. Timing

We have observed that there is a point at which a social movement incorporates the vast majority of people in a community. These movements are very powerful and their power may be expressed through many spheres. Traditionally, social power was viewed as evolving to political power. Through our experience, we have seen that this social power may be directly expressed through market functions.

Our start-ups are fueled less intensely by financial capital and more through the transformation of the underlying social capital. Our companies are built, at their core, to extend, reinforce, and amplify the values represented in the community and the social movement. Our flour mill does well precisely when the values of the local food movement are expressed as consumer behavior. We mirror these values and are supported by them.

Of course, social movements take a long time to gain hold. Finding the right social movement in a specific community with an aligned business model at the right time is the art of this development method and takes patience and experience.

For reference, here are some illustrative timelines for two social movements we have helped develop through community building companies.

Microcredit:

1983 Grameen Bank Founded

2005 UN Year of Microcredit

2006 UEF founded – We initiate investing in microcredit

Mohammad Yunus wins Nobel Prize for microcredit

2014 100 million worldwide borrowers, many public companies

Food System:

1970 First Earth Day

2002 USDA Organic Food Designation Enacted

2010 First Lady Michelle Obama launches healthy food initiative, Let's Move!

2015 Cairnspring Mills established to commercialize healthy, local, and fresh flour

The key here is to acknowledge that movements such as local food and microcredit do not just represent trends. Local food represents the common need for healthy food and unstructured activity, while microcredit represents basic access to capital and human empowerment in poor communities. In these examples, communities have taken into their own hands the instinct and means of change.

One indicator that a movement is ready for development in the commercial sphere is indicated when the movement ceases to be perceived as political within the relevant communities. While movements remain politicized, there is insufficient agreement; when the community itself is split in its support, this method of commercial development is doomed at the outset. On the other hand, it was obvious in the case of both microcredit and local food, that virtually everyone in the local communities agreed with the underlying premise. When the commercial, values-aligned community business models were tested, they were able to attract nearly unanimous support.

CLIENT NOTICE, PLAN SPONSOR BILL OF RIGHTS, AND CODE OF CONDUCT

Sample Health Rosetta Client Notice

Congratulations! We're excited you've decided to work with a Health Rosetta Certified Benefits Professional. The Health Rosetta ecosystem's mission is to help group benefits purchasers sustainably reduce health benefits costs and provide better care for their employees. We maintain the Health Rosetta, an expert sourced blueprint for wisely purchasing benefits sourced from the highest-performing benefits purchasers and experts everywhere.

A primary goal of Health Rosetta certification programs is to help benefits purchasers reduce your spending while improving the quality of care your plan members receive. This notice is to help you understand what to expect while working with a Health Rosetta advisor.

What to Expect?

One of our core principles is that higher transparency, trust, and integrity in the purchasing process improves the quality of benefits-purchasing decisions. To facilitate this, HRI certified professionals commit in our agreement with them to adhere to certain specific practices.

- Only make changes that have been shown to improve care while improving your costs AND your employees' costs. No more choosing between hurting you or hurting your employees.
- Review this notice with you to set expectations.
- Fully and meaningfully disclose their compensation in writing.
- Think, plan, and act in your long-term interests, including completing 3-5-year strategic plans.
- Adhere to the HR Code of Conduct you should have received with this notice.
- Adhere to the HR. Plan Sponsor Bill of Rights you should have receive with this notice.

These practices significantly differentiate both certified professionals and their design, purchasing, and management process from the highly-conflicted, opaque status quo process. To maintain the quality of HRI certification programs, they'll ask you to sign this notice and a couple other documents throughout the purchasing process.

How the Health Rosetta Ecosystem and Certification Benefit You

You'll likely benefit both directly and indirectly as a result of working with a HRI-certified benefits professional. Here are a couple of the main ways.

- Higher-value benefits – You should experience better returns in the form of sustainably lower costs and higher quality care within the next 12 months. While we can't promise specifics, as this varies on many factors, Health Rosetta components implemented by other employers have sustainably reduced their spending by 10-40% per year.

- Access to a deep ecosystem of solutions and best practices – Our health care system is in the early days of a dramatic transformation, with many new innovative approaches. This makes it difficult for you and most advisors to easily navigate. Certified professionals have access to other certified people, industry leading experts, the Health Rosetta blueprint, and other community resources to sift through this, improving the likelihood that design changes, programs, technologies, and services you implement are appropriate and likely to work.
- Learning from others – The education and other resources we make available for certified professionals are based on the real-life experience of other purchasers, not theory. We actively cultivate shared learning to keep us abreast. We maintain a network of more than 3,500 experts and high national visibility to create a hivemind for identifying the best approaches. See just a few of our collaborators at healthrosetta.org/whowe-are/.

We have high expectations for certified professionals and work to attract those seeking to go above and beyond them. However, if you feel your certified professional is not meeting your needs, discuss with them or contact us directly at employers@healthrosetta.org. We're happy to help. You can find more resources, our book, *The CEO's Guide to Restoring the American Dream*, and subscribe to updates and education at healthrosetta.org.

From Dave, Sean, and the entire Health Rosetta team, we'd like to thank you for choosing to work with a HR-Certified Professional.

Health Rosetta Plan Sponsor Bill of Rights

1. Service Agreement Fiduciary Duty Protection

You have the right to ensure that your obligations as your plan's sponsor, administrator, and fiduciary are protected and enhanced in your service agreement.

2. *Transparent Relationships & Conflict Disclosure*

You have the right to expect transparency, including disclosure of conflicts, in financial dealings between you and your broker, advisor, or consultant, carriers, and vendors.

3. *Independence*

You have the right to ensure those financial dealings do not compromise your fiduciary responsibility and the independence of the advice you receive.

4. *Access to all options*

You have the right to receive information about the full range of options available to you, not just those that preserve or optimize your representative's income or plan administrator's revenue.

5. *Independent Review*

You have the right to an unbiased, independent review of all pertinent market options in an impartial manner, not just those that preserve or optimize your representative's income or plan administrator's revenue.

6. *Comprehensive Reporting*

You have the right to receive comprehensive reporting of your costs, and the potential drivers of those costs.

7. *Answers to Questions*

You have the right to receive answers to your questions, with no cloaking of responses with HIPAA Privacy and other "confidentiality" curtains.

8. *Effective Adjudication*

You have the right to expect those you hire to adjudicate benefits to give their best effort to identifying inappropriate and grossly inflated charges before they issue payment.

9. Access to data

You have the right to your data and should agree upon this requirement prior to execution of any vendor agreement.

10. Complete reporting

You have the right to receive complete service and outcome reporting from each of your vendors, including all fees associated with services rendered.

Health Rosetta Benefits Advisor Code of Conduct

Good for employees and employers

We resolve to only implement programs and solutions that seek to improve the plan sponsor's bottom line, the plan member's bottom line, and, most importantly, the plan member's health.

Programs should do no harm

We resolve that brokers, consultants, and advisors should do no harm to employee health, corporate integrity, or employee/ employer finances. Instead, we will endeavor to support employee well-being for our customers, their employees, and all program constituents.

Employee Benefits and Harm Avoidance

We will only recommend implementing programs with/ for employees rather than to them, and will focus on promoting responsible practices for the health plans we serve.

Our choices of programs and strategies shall always prioritize best outcomes at the lowest cost, in that order, with a strong focus on the responsibility that an employer should provide affordable coverage for their employees while respecting the financial integrity of the business.

Respect for Corporate Integrity and Employee Privacy

We will not share employee-identifiable data with employers and will ensure that all protected health information (PHI) adheres to HIPAA regulations and any other applicable laws.

Commitment to Transparency

Our focus shall be to bring transparency to all levels of health care financing. From how we get paid to how insurance companies and PBMs get paid to how providers get paid.

Commitment to Valid Outcomes

Measurement of contractual language and outcomes reporting will be transparent and plausible. The end goal is to improve outcomes and quality of care while lowering costs, and the ability to do this shall be measured and reported on in a valid, consistent, and accountable format.

SAMPLE COMPENSATION DISCLOSURE FORM

The following is a sample broker compensation disclosure form to help you improve your benefits purchasing process. The status quo is rife with conflicts of interest stemming from undisclosed compensation arrangements. This prevents benefits purchasers from making the most informed and intelligent purchasing decisions. We've found that the first step toward high-performance benefits is disclosure of incentives to minimize conflicts, create transparency, and increase trust in your advisors and process.

Calculation of Fees

In general, each fee should be calculated in one of five ways.

1. **Premium based.** Fees are based on the amount of premium for each line of coverage. This is normally expressed as a predetermined percentage.
2. **Claims-based.** Fees are based on the $ amount or number of claims in the plan and generally are expressed as percentages or aggregate per-claim fees for the period.
3. **Per eligible employee or per member per month (PEPM or PMPM).** Fees are based on the number of eligible employees or actual members in the plan.

4. **Transaction-based**. Fees are based on the execution of a particular plan service or transaction.
5. **Flat rate**. Fees are a fixed charge that does not vary, regardless of plan size

You can also access a regularly updated digital version of this firm on the Health Rosetta's website (healthrosetta.org).

HEALTH ROSETTA BENEFITS REPRESENTATIVE COMPENSATION DISCLOSURE FORM

Advisor: _____   Client: _____   Period: _____

Background

A key element of the Health Rosetta's mission is to help benefits purchasers build transparent, trusted relationships with benefits advisors. These relationships are critical to an effective benefits-purchasing process, particularly in today's world of skyrocketing health care costs and limited ability to push those costs on employees. This form is one resource to help you.

Advisor compensation is a small portion of total spend, but the right one can guide the way to dramatic improvements in your plan costs and quality. The total amount shouldn't be the primary focus. Instead, it should help build trust and identify potential conflicts.

High-value, forward-leaning advisors are worth their weight in gold. Plus, the strategies they use typically improve your bottom line, reduce your employees' out-of-pocket spending, and improve the quality of care they receive. Think of it this way:

Would you rather pay four percent to an advisor who reduces total spending by 15 percent or two percent to one who "negotiates" a 15 percent increase down to a seven percent increase? For every 100 employ-

ees on an average plan, you'd save $247,220 in year 1 and $1.2 million in 5 years (net of the higher compensation).

Unwillingness to disclose compensation is typically a red flag that recommendations may not align with your interests. The benefits world often has undisclosed conflicts and incentives that make intelligent purchasing decisions difficult. To help you get around this, we've created a free guide for selecting high-value advisors.

Contact us at healthrosetta.org to learn more about improving the cost and quality of your health plan, about Certified Advisors, and about how we help benefits purchasers. A special thanks to Eric Krieg at Risk International Benefits Advisory, David Contorno at E Powered Benefits, Josh Jeffries at Arkin Youngentob Associates, and Tom Emerick at Edison Health for helping create this form. Each is a worth-their-weight-in-gold type.

Overview of Services Provided

Some fees may be estimates and will vary throughout the course of the year. However, the variance should not be significant (unless something significant/unplanned happens).

Service Provided	External Vendor	Cost/ Fee for Service	Compensation Type	Total Compensation
Core Consulting Services				
Pharmacy Consulting Services				
Actuarial Services				
Compliance Services				
Wellness Consulting				
Claims Audit				
Data Analytics and Clinical Services				

Communications				
Decision Support Services and Transparency Resources				
Benefits Administration				
Total Projected Annual Costs				

Expected Financial Compensation from External Vendors

Category	Vendor	Effective Date	Compensation Type	Total Compensation
Medical				
Rx				
Dental				
Vision				
Stop loss				
EAP				
FSA				
Group Life				
AD&D				
LT Disability				
ST Disability				
Cancer				
Critical Illness				
Wellness				
Disease Mgmt.				
Broker Fee				
Other				
Total				

Are any compensation multipliers or other bonuses applicable to the above categories of compensation?
☐ Yes (please describe below)   ☐ No

If yes, are they included in the above dollar amounts?
☐ Yes   ☐ No

Do you or your firm accept any non-account specific financial compensation from any products, services, or vendors you're recommending, including, but not limited to, contingent or bonus commissions, override or retention bonuses, and backend commissions.
☐ Yes (please describe below)   ☐ No

Do you or your firm have any other financial or non-financial compensation, potential conflicts of interest, or incentives related to products, services, or vendors you're recommending, including, but not limited to, ownership, equity stakes, revenue/profit sharing, GPO/coalition participation, preferred vendor panels, conferences or trips, or personal relationships.
☐ Yes (please describe below)   ☐ No

Are there any potential reasons that could cause costs of services or compensation to vary more than 10 percent from the above projections?
☐ Yes (please describe below)   ☐ No

Please describe details related to any questions to which you answered yes above, including the specific, expected, or estimated dollar value. Attach additional pages if necessary.

Total Expected Compensation

Consulting Services	
Compensation from External Vendors	
Cost of Services from External Vendors	

Advisor

I certify that to the best of my knowledge the above is a complete and meaningful disclosure of my firm's entire compensation.

Client

I acknowledge that the signed Certified Advisor has presented and adequately reviewed the above disclosures.

Name: _____

Entity: _____

Title: _____

Signed:_____

Date _____

Name: _____

Entity: _____

Title: _____

Signed: _____

Date _____

HEALTH ROSETTA PRINCIPLES

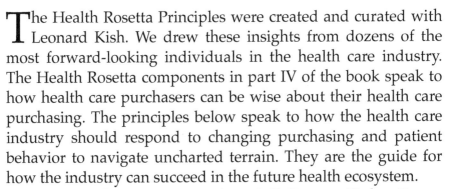

The Health Rosetta Principles were created and curated with Leonard Kish. We drew these insights from dozens of the most forward-looking individuals in the health care industry. The Health Rosetta components in part IV of the book speak to how health care purchasers can be wise about their health care purchasing. The principles below speak to how the health care industry should respond to changing purchasing and patient behavior to navigate uncharted terrain. They are the guide for how the industry can succeed in the future health ecosystem.

Leading thinkers ranging from Bill Gates to Esther Dyson have written essays on specific principles that we invite you to read at healthrosetta.org/health-rosetta-principles. The essays expand on each principle to make them more actionable. In the open-source spirit of the Health Rosetta, we invite others to contribute their essays to advance the cause.

A New Medical Science

1. *A New Paradigm* – A new social, psychological, biological, and information-driven medical science is emerging that will better understand a person's environmental context and its relationship with disease. It's precision medicine but more, using sensors and networks to better predict and prevent as well as treat

the root causes of disease. No vision of the future of medicine can be complete or even competent if it doesn't recognize these new sources of information and the power of patient engagement.

2. *Open source and open knowledge* – Open source, open APIs, open data, and open knowledge (such as wikis) will become central to defining a common architecture to support this new science. These are modern versions of peer review.

3. *Nonclinical determinants of outcomes* – To improve care and reduce costs with this new science, we must focus on what drives 80 percent of outcomes, the nonclinical factors, which include social, economic, and psychological determinants of health.

4. *Cross-disciplinary collaboration* – Cross-disciplinary collaboration and sharing of research data will be a requirement to accelerate new discoveries.

5. *Evidence-based understanding of what works* – This new science will arrive at an evidence-based understanding of what works through a great wealth of shared longitudinal health data captured through mobile devices, sensors, and health records. It must be mindful of the concept of transforming data to actionable information, knowledge, and wisdom.

6. *Understanding the personome* – The new medical science will focus on understanding the personome. "The influence of the unique circumstances of the person—the personome—is just as powerful as the impact of that individual's genome, proteome, pharmacogenome, metabolome, and epigenome."[185]

Openness Drives Effective Action

7. *Individual choice* – Individuals have the right to make choices and control their health destiny with the best information available.

8. *Open access to information* – Open access to information will enable individuals to make the best decisions and become well-informed individuals, particularly when curated and contextualized by clinicians.

9. *Openness and privacy are not in conflict* – Openness and privacy are not in conflict with the right kinds of identity, consent, and data-control mechanisms in place.

10. *A required culture change* – This openness will come with a required culture change. We must release information in order to ensure high-quality information and code. In software, Linus' Law states, "Given enough eyeballs, all bugs are shallow." Keeping information sealed until it is perfect will mean we miss opportunities to improve the data and fix the system.

Economics and Transparency

11. *Information asymmetries* – Information asymmetries lead to inefficient systems and suboptimal outcomes. Access to life-saving, taxpayer-supported research must be open.

12. *Social determinants of health* – Health and wealth are tightly linked. Eventually, poor financial health will negatively impact overall health.

13. *Cost as comorbidity* – The cost of care can be a comorbidity. By ignoring costs in clinical decisions, conditions can worsen as financial stress may drive individuals to choose not to follow a plan of care because it is too expensive.

14. *Individual's right to know the cost of care* – Individuals have the right to know how much care will cost before receiving care, whether that cost is out-of-pocket or covered. When there is unpredictable complexity (not caused by medical error, which shouldn't be charged for at all), individuals should be informed of the most likely ranges.

15. *Personal responsibility* – Individuals have personal responsibility to manage their lives along with their care.

Relationships and Peer-to-Peer Networks Will Become Central

16. *Communication as medical instrument* – The most important "medical instrument" is communication. Communications drive actions, build relationships, and create trust.
17. *Data liquidity for improving health* – Exchange of personal health data will become enabled via decentralized Peer-to-Peer (P2P) networks and "HIEs of 1." These P2P exchanges will improve health literacy, healthy action, and a functioning health economy.
18. *P2P networked conversations* – P2P networked conversations will empower new ways of better organizing health, allowing individuals to "organize without organizations" (h/t Clay Shirky) for better care.
19. *Individuals and health research* – Verifiable but deidentified, opt-in health data will become part of a unified view for research and risk assessment. Individuals will have the choice to contribute.

New Intelligence

20. *Cognification* – To "Cognify" (h/t Kevin Kelly) is to instill intelligence into something. Medical knowledge will increasingly be "cognified" into the IoT as much of the world around us is made "smart" and data-aware. This is good and will free people to care for themselves where and when they choose.
21. *Feedback* – All feedback has utility. Whether the news is good or bad, opinions that become known are a source for improvement and competitiveness.

Community-driven Health

22. *Stewarding social and economic factors* – True health system leadership comes from not just being stewards of hospitals

and clinics but stewarding social and economic factors and the physical environment of a community, which account for half of outcomes.

23. *Partnering for community health* – Assessing community health needs and adopting strategies to address those needs will provide hospitals with a valuable opportunity for community partnerships to identify strategies for improving health, quality of life, and the community's vitality.

24. *Building health literacy and community* – Health care organizations that aggressively promote health literacy will build community capacity in addressing health issues. This may mean enabling and curating others in the community to reach everyone.

25. *Health and financial literacy* – Start by teaching medicine and psychological self-awareness and resilience to kids. Health education should include the "medicine" we consume every day (i.e., food). Insurance/benefits literacy should be included in schools' financial literacy courses.

26. *School lunches* – School lunches are an access point of great power: they reinforce or remove the unhealthy products we consume.

27. *"Let food be thy medicine"* – Hippocrates said, "Let food be thy medicine and medicine be thy food." Individuals are "poisoning" themselves with the food they eat, largely without knowing it.

28. *"Walking is man's best medicine."* – Hippocrates also said, "Walking is man's best medicine." Communities and workplaces that make it easy to walk and be active can gain an advantage over the status quo.

29. *Health care waste: A bandit stealing from our future* –Health care is breaking U.S. schools. Money once directed to education is getting gobbled up by health care's hyperinflation, exacerbating the problem that kids don't learn enough about health, nutrition, finance, or any of the things that lead to healthy, long lives.

New Choices for Individuals and Care Teams

30. *Health isn't limited to the clinic* – Health is not the limited time individuals spend in clinics. What happens in the other 99+ percent of their life has the greater impact on an individual's overall well-being.

31. *Better choices through motivation* – We will learn how to rapidly enable better choices through motivation, tools, and access to better choices and lifestyles. Each individual will respond differently, requiring a whole new level of personalization.

32. *Understanding motivations and habit change* – People are complicated with both innate drives and ingrained habits that work against long-term health. The psychology of understanding these motivations and habits is critical to success in achieving better health.

33. *Wisdom of the individual* – People will make incredibly smart decisions when they understand the true risks and choices.

34. *Mental health* – Mental health is an equal component of a person's overall health. Mental health directly impacts our physical health and our ability to recover from disease or medical interventions. Therefore, mental health needs to be deliberately and systematically integrated into the general health care system.

35. *Nutritional and environmental causes of disease* – Open information and research are needed to understand the nutritional and environmental causes of disease.

36. *Unhealthy food* – Foods that are devoid of nutrition are the tobacco of this generation.

37. *Optimizing health* – We have defined sick care very well: what happens when things go wrong and how to correct them. We have very little understanding of how to keep things going right, how to get people back on track when they go off the rails, or how to continually optimize health. Innovations in research are changing this; new entrants will figure out how to enable it.

38. *Preventing the need for care* – Systems will be designed so individuals can stay healthy, take as few drugs and have as few procedures as possible, and avoid the system as much as possible by engaging in self-care.

39. *Embracing the "flat world" of care* – The emergence of a flat world opens new avenues to innovation around what has worked in other cultures. We have the opportunity to learn to be open to ways of health care that originate outside our borders, particularly those that are more appropriate to the underserved.

Individuals and Engagement

40. *Inclusivity with individuals and caregivers* – Individuals and their everyday caregivers are the greatest untapped sources of information, knowledge, and motivation. Empowering them to work together will optimize care.

41. *Experience had a "Triple Aim" too* – The effectiveness of engagement is tightly aligned with how convenient it is; how easily it integrates with where we live, work, and play; and how culturally relevant and cost-effective it is.

42. *Leveling the playing field* – Engagement and empowerment are different. Individuals are often most engaged, but least empowered. Putting individuals and clinicians on the same level will improve care.

43. *"Patient engagement" is backwards* – "Patient engagement" is valuable but backwards. Individuals need the health system to be engaged with them and regularly, not just during visits.

44. *"Individual-centered" engagement* – An engaged individual is very different from "patient engagement" (h/t Gilles Frydman). One is individual-centered, one is health system-centered. Achieving full health is the goal, not engaging with the health system.

45. *Engagement for avoiding the health system* – An individual can be engaged with their own health without entering the health system at all (h/t Hugo Campos), and this is a good thing.

New Economics

46. *Choose wisely* – Oftentimes, less is more.
47. *Prevention* – Oftentimes, early is better than late.
48. *Overtreatment* – Overtreatment is one of health care's greatest challenges. In many cases, no treatment is much better than treatment.
49. *Sustainability* – A system that profits more from people with "problems" than those without and has a default set at "treat more" is destined to collapse due to its inherent unsustainability.
50. *Evidence-based care delivery* – Driven by individual's access to information and, informed by statistics, treatment will become better aligned with science.
51. *Empowering a patient to make rational economic choices* – Individuals enter the health care system to get measurements; to be diagnosed; and to seek answers and, when appropriate, treatment. Individuals who can will increasingly seek alternatives outside of expensive, inconvenient care centers. This will drive positive overall change in the health system.

New Education

52. *Scaling medical education for the future* – Medical education will be made continuous, engaging, and scalable in the age of increasing clinical demands and limited work hours.
53. *New approaches to learning* – Medical educators will make thoughtful use of technology and learning design. Those who excel will learn how Massive Open Online Courses (MOOCs), community engagement, social media, simulation, and virtual reality can enhance medical education.
54. *Harnessing the data deluge* – The flood of new medical information is impossible for any one person to stay on top of. Physicians and other care providers will be enabled by better systems for filtering what's valuable for an individual's care.

55. *Rapid evolution* – Effective medical education must and will evolve rapidly to focus on care delivery and the use of digital tools in care delivery.

56. *Physician as community manager* – Medical education will recognize that, because only 10–20 percent of health outcomes are driven by clinical care, physicians must also be stewards of community transformation, entering into multidisciplinary alliances.

New Data Ownership Rights

57. *Individual Rights* – An individual's access to and management of data about him/herself is a fundamental human and property right. Why is it easier to have your medical data hacked than for you to get access to it? (h/t Eric Topol)

58. *Monopolies* – Monopolies on medical knowledge and information are unethical.

59. *Single Patient Record* – Now that all information can be connected all the time, there should be only one record of health data that comes from an individual, controlled by the individual. Problems with HIPAA and "information blocking" are symptoms of a broken, pre-Internet, paper-driven era.

60. *Property Rights in a Distributed System* – Platforms will be developed to enable transactions around health data property that are decentralized, yet able to focus on the individual in an instant. Be prepared.

61. *Patients' Right to Data About Them* – Individuals have a right to any data that comes from measuring an internal state of their body, including from medical devices.

62. *Immediacy of Access to Health Data* – People have literally died, waiting for their lab data. Lab and other data should be made accessible to the individuals as soon as it is available.

63. *Data Doesn't Cause Medical Harm* – Medical regulations exist to protect individuals from medical harm. Data, ideas, and information in the hands of individuals cause no medical harm.

64. *Safe Access to Data Without a Doctor's Permission* – Individuals should have access to metrics and analysis about their own body without a doctor's permission as long as that access poses no significant medical risk.

65. *Right to Privacy* – Individuals have a right to health data privacy and only they or their legal agent can give permission for sharing their data.

66. *Health Information Anti-Discrimination* – Health data collected about an individual cannot be used to determine a person's access to capital (via credit ratings), employment, education, housing, or health care services. This will be legislated and ensured by new technologies.

New Roles and Relationships for Providers

67. *Misaligned Incentives* – Misaligned reimbursement schemes have impaired providers from doing the primary job of healing and have often robbed them of their humanity. Paying for value will help them reverse course.

68. *Enlightened Providers Partner with Patients* – The enlightened clinicians who embrace these guiding principles will gain a powerful competitive advantage by partnering with patients who have taken responsibility for their own care.

69. *Maintain Trust in Health Professionals* – Nurses, doctors, and pharmacists are among the most trusted professionals; they need to respect this trust and continue to earn it by influencing patients only for the patients' good.

70. *Whole-Person View of Health* – World class care teams require a holistic view of a person's complete health, which includes their mental health as well as their physical health.

71. *Embracing the Science of Behavior Change* – Relationships fuel behavior change (both positive and negative); motivation, triggers, and ease of action are keys to enabling that change.

72. *The Importance of Relationships* – Aim to motivate, teach, consult, and enable. Clinicians cannot expect participation in a care plan (i.e., "adherence") without mutual understanding. Recognize

that when an individual is not incapacitated, they are in control of whether they fill prescriptions, follow a care plan, etc.

73. *Health Care Extends Beyond the Walls of the Clinic* – The best care is and will be collaborative beyond the walls of any one institution. Just as "the smartest people work for someone else," the smartest providers practice outside of one clinic or hospital. The smartest provider may, in fact, be a collective, or the crowd. New ways to open communications will drive better care.

74. *Flipping the Clinic* – Many times, the best place for interaction between the clinician and an individual isn't at the clinic. We can flip the clinic. Much of what has been done at a clinic visit can be done more effectively in the comfort of an individual's home via email and other digital tools or in social settings such as churches or community organizations.

75. *Embracing Data to Deliver Better Care* – The most relevant providers will be conversant with data analytics and tools. They will be experts in care delivery, not just diagnostics and traditional medical science.

A New Competition in Life Science & MedTech

76. *Embracing the New Science*– Tomorrow's leaders will redesign research and development to capitalize on new science dynamics and mobile technologies.

77. *Embracing New Partnerships*– New and nonobvious partnerships will need to be forged to ensure leadership in the future. Alliances with health tech and consumer health Internet companies will be as important as alliances with academic medical centers have been in the past.

78. *Broadening the Value of Post Research Relationships* – Post-trial relationships with individuals will allow cocreation and insights not possible before. That is a largely untapped opportunity. ResearchKit is just the beginning.

79. *Openness to Engagement* – The individual's relationship to a device or therapeutic may be as profound as their relationship to their doctor, or more so. Be available and open to such engagement to make improvements.

New Health Plans, New Health Benefits

80. *Fee for Service Is Dying* –Transition now in every way you can.
81. *The Dirty Secret of Health Plans* – The dirty secret of health plans is that higher care costs have, counterintuitively, led to greater profits for the plans. This is changing. Winning health plans will capitalize on the opportunity to fundamentally rethink plan design to be optimized for the fee-for-value era.
82. *Catalyzing Patient Engagement* – Catalyzing patient engagement will lead to better care and a more competitive offering.
83. *The Next Dirty Secret* – The next dirty secret of health plans is that they are money managers. The longer they hold onto money, the more they make.
84. *Investing in Members' Financial Security* – Rather than reflexively denying claims and building up a mountain of ill will, insurance companies should invest resources in protecting their member's financial security.
85. *The "Negaclaim"* – Customers will, in effect, "self-deny" their own claims. A new metric for success is the "Negaclaim"—an unnecessary claim avoided. This isn't about denying care. Just as energy consumers aren't interested in kilowatt hours, individuals aren't interested in health claims—they want health restored and diseases prevented.
86. *True Informed Consent* – When individuals are fully educated on the trade-offs associated with interventions, they generally choose the less invasive approach.
87. *"Essential Access," the Corollary to "Essential Benefits"*—The ACA defined "essential benefits" but there will be a corollary about rights to "essential access" as part of coverage. Any modern health plan offering will include virtual visits, transparent price info, updated provider directory, same-day

e-mail response, next-day test results, etc.—all eminently doable with today's modern technology.

88. *Rethinking Benefits Design and Procurement* – CFOs & CEOs are failing in their fiduciary responsibility by being overly passive in how they procure health benefits, the second or third biggest expense after payroll. A rethought health care purchasing plan drives direct financial returns, but, most importantly, enables your valued employees to do what they desire—realize their full potential. Elements are defined at healthrosetta.org.

89. *Aligning Laboratory Testing and Genomics* – Genomics and proteomics information and testing will be key components of personalized medications, tailored to provide the best dose/response relationship in each patient. Because of their importance, these tests and genomic information must be covered by health plans and insurance.

New Health System

90. *Transitioning Care Beyond the Walls of the Clinic* – Hospitals have provided amazing service for the last 100 years, but location is becoming less important for health care. Care can happen almost anywhere at lower cost. What conditions hospitals treat, and how hospitals serve their communities will dramatically change over the coming decades.

91. *Reimagining Technology in the Fee-for-Value Era* – Health systems' technology procurement process must be up to the task. Systems grown and optimized for the waning fee-for-service era often have the polar opposite design to what will optimize the fee-for-value era. Virtually every new health care delivery organization that is outperforming on Triple Aim objectives has deployed new technology reimagined.

92. *Focusing on Communication over Billing* – Outside of health care, millions of organizations have reformulated how they interact with their ultimate customers with better communications tools. Next generation health care leaders understand that tools will focus on communication over billing.

93. *Borrowing a Page from the Newspaper Industry* –Newspaper executives dismissed an array of new asymmetric competitors including eBay, Craigslist, Monster.com, Cars.com, Facebook, Groupon, ESPN, CBS Marketwatch and more who stole advertising, media consumption, or both. Health system executives are doing the same thing today, and the issue is the same: how valuable content will be delivered in the future. The content is different, but the issue of distribution is the same.

94. *The "Forgotten" Fourth Aim* – Winning health care delivery organizations recognize that the Quadruple Aim will deliver sustainable success. The "forgotten aim" is a better experience for the health professional, which leads to a better experience and better outcomes for patients. Layering more bureaucracy on top of an already overburdened clinical team ignores that the underlying processes are frequently underperforming and that a bad professional experience negatively impacts patient outcomes.

95. *Unshackling Innovation* – Health care organizations wanting to reinvent can harness new opportunities by unshackling their smart, innovative team members and outside thinkers to reinvent their organizations for the next 100 years. Those that enable their customers will emerge as the leaders for the next 100 years.

WHY DOCTORS ARE RUNNING OUT OF EMPATHY

Those not enmeshed in health care typically are unaware of how dramatically things have changed for physicians. The majority of physicians will no longer recommend their profession to their children. Of course, that is the tip of the iceberg. As mentioned earlier in the book, there are record levels of burnout and even suicide for physicians. The only silver lining is that the experience in far too many hospitals is so appalling for physicians that it leaves many physicians no choice but to either leave the profession or be leaders in the next 100 years of modern medicine. Dr. Mohseni is a good example. He left the toxic work environment and is working on a new health care delivery model to address a large unmet need. The following essay beautifully captures the problems that are far too frequent in hospitals today.

As health care is transformed and hospitals either reinvent themselves and their culture or they perish, we shouldn't over-sentimentalize today's hospital environment. It's important that we understand that the under-performance on health outcomes in our status quo health care system is only matched by how much physicians, nurses and other clinicians are frequently victimized in hospitals.

Inside the "sickness-billing industrial complex"

By Alex Mohseni, MD

Walking up to the door of the waiting room, I knew what lay behind it. The gnawing torment would start the day before, or sometimes two days prior. Three parts nausea, two parts dread, and a dash of anxiety — the recipe was always the same. Just add an organic grass-fed doctor, and you have yourself a nice little snack for the healthcare system to chew up and unceremoniously spit out.

This is my story: a successful emergency medicine physician by external parameters, but internally strained. The person who came out of residency—a supremely confident physician ready to take on the world—would never recognize himself 11 years later. My experiences in our healthcare system transformed me, and my story is not unique. There is a sickness that permeates our medical providers within our healthcare system: it is as easy to catch as influenza and as hard to treat.

But before we diagnose this sickness, I would like to describe the context within which we work, this so-called "healthcare system." I find the phrase "healthcare system" difficult to write, because it is an inaccurate representation of what it purports to describe. If we take the word "healthcare" to mean the mishmash of hospitals, doctors, insurance companies, and vendors that profit from our physical and mental maladies, then perhaps it would be more accurate to call it "sickness-billing." It is truly "sickness" rather than "health" that the industry focuses on, and "billing" rather than "care" on which it spends the better portion of its time. And if we take the word "system" to mean an organized set of people working together for a common goal, and if one has ever spent a day in a hospital, then one recognizes that the word "ataxia" better communicates the reality of the experience. "Ataxia" is a medical term we use to describe the inability of a person to move their body in a coordinated way.

But "ataxia" may be too obscure, so I'll use the term "industrial complex"—just think of the patients as our industry's widgets.

This sickness-billing industrial complex, or SBIC—our healthcare system's true identity—is an uncoordinated amalgam of special interests profiting from a series of unintended consequences of poorly designed policies. So how did we go from "healthcare" to the SBIC? What happened in the last 20 to 30 years? Here is my version of the story.

Government food policies, such as the subsidization of corn and the promotion of sugar- and carbohydrate-rich foods as "low-fat" alternatives, resulted in a massive increase in calorie-dense, nutrient-poor, and highly processed "foods" in our diet (corn syrup, other sugars, refined wheat, etc.). In addition, societal expectations of portion size and taste transformed as well. These dietary changes have led to dramatic increases in obesity, diabetes, heart disease, cancer, and rates in the United States. The costs borne by Medicare and insurance companies consequently swelled, producing a strained "system" unprepared to handle the increasing need for preventive care. In response to rapidly rising costs, Medicare (to which most insurance companies look for guidance) created a growing number of obstacles to reimbursing doctors and hospitals, and all payers followed suit. These obstacles started as documentation-focused rules, requiring doctors to record a certain number of data points for each medical visit, otherwise reducing reimbursement. This is why your doctor, during your visit for an ankle sprain, may ask if you have had any constipation, vaginal bleeding, or ringing in your ears.

Doctors—often slow, but never dumb—adapted to the new rules, and learned how to recover their lost revenue by spending extra time asking unnecessary questions and documenting endless nonsense in patients' medical charts. Medicare created a game and the doctors learned how to play it, to the detriment of patients. Eventually Medicare piled on even more barriers, which they termed Core Measures. Of course, Medicare couldn't call these things "barriers to paying doctors and hospitals," so it spun the changes as a switch to "value-based care." The problem was, most of the parameters on which it was basing "value" were questionable, with little basis in the scientific literature. Most doctors saw the parameters for what they were: barriers to reimbursement.

Sure enough, the Core Measure program went awry and led to a variety of unintended consequences. At a particular hospital emergency room where I worked, it was decided that all patients who had the remotest possibility of having pneumonia upon their initial evaluation in triage were to be given a dose of antibiotics by mouth immediately, because Medicare had decided that getting antibiotics within six hours of arrival to the ER was a measure of quality. Some patients ended up getting antibiotics they did not need, while others needed IV antibiotics but had just received oral instead. In order to meet our "quality" goal, we were practicing bad medicine.

After doctors and hospitals mastered the Core Measure game, Medicare created yet more games, represented by a seemingly never-ending litany of acronyms that read like a Sesame Street song, from "PQRS," to "MIPS," to "MACRA." These new programs were of such complexity that many doctors were faced with three stark choices: 1) spend hundreds of hours trying to learn and adapt to the new rules, 2) sell their practice to a hospital or much larger group (an entity with the resources to hire a consultant to help them figure out how to play the game), or 3) give up and just accept the significantly lower payment.

Sadly, many physicians have opted to sell their practices and give up their autonomy to a corporate entity. This is a major loss to our communities, as independent physician practices are some of the last refuges against the corporate practice of medicine. Just as sad are those doctors who try to stay afloat in the sea of acronyms, barely keeping their heads above water and seeing patients ever more hastily, with less patient face-to-face time, more stress, more rushing, more mistakes, and more frustration—all of which may lead to a dangerous decrease in the physician's capacity for empathy.

None of these new Medicare programs will work to solve the problems within our sickness-billing industrial complex, because we are not dealing with the core fundamental issues: we're treating sickness instead of fostering health, we focus on billing instead of care, and we are completely ataxic (uncoordinated). We have a very unhealthy population gorging themselves on sugar-rich foods, developing preventable diseases, like type 2 diabetes, with very expensive complications (kidney failure, heart attack, stroke, blindness, etc.), and clinging to unrealistic expectations that doctors and medicines can work miracles to reverse the impact of years of horrendous nutrition. Meanwhile, we have doctors being coerced to spend a majority of their time figuring out how to play documentation games instead of engaging patients in real health-oriented change.

In 2006, within this context of the SBIC, came a fresh, young, eager new emergency medicine doctor. I truly loved learning about and practicing medicine when I began my career. It was exhilarating—the tight-knit teams of nurses, techs, secretaries, physician assistants, and doctors dealing with the chaos of endless streams of patients, with time pressure, challenging problem-solving, and quick decision-making. Great teamwork, amazing saves, and warm appreciation from patients were the norm.

Then, in my second year, came my first lawsuit as an attending ("attending" refers to doctors working without supervision, having graduated from residency). It was a case I remembered with photographic precision, because it was one of my most intense. A patient who'd been seen by several previous physicians was admitted for a complaint with a very atypical presentation. The patient later crashed during my shift and my team and I did our best to save him. I remember having a very heartfelt, warm, and sad moment with his family at his bedside before we sent him via helicopter for an emergency surgery that we could not perform at our hospital. Unfortunately, he did not survive. That night, although very saddened about this gentleman's death, I was proud of my team's effort. In court I recounted the scene of the woman from the blood bank running her fastest into the ER with several units of O-negative blood in her hand, knowing that every second counted; every single person was doing everything he or she could to save this man's life.

I felt like a leader of heroes. Yet, we were sued, and treated like criminals. To be sued when you've done something egregiously wrong is understandable. But when you're proud of your own and your team's effort, skill, and decision-making, and cannot imagine what you could have done better, being sued is demoralizing and discombobulating. To be sued when you remember standing by the patient's bedside, your own eyes welling up with tears, because you are a human being who feels the suffering of those around you...

"I did my best. I did what I thought was right. Every medical decision and intervention I made was correct. And somebody hates me so much, they want to ruin my life and end my career. Somebody thinks I did everything wrong. Somebody thinks I am evil." Such was the narrative swimming in my mind for the two years this case was active. Sleepless nights. Stressful shifts. Two years of self-doubt chipping away at my confidence and pride.

When self-doubt takes a foothold in an emergency medicine physician, it is poison. The hallmark of a great ER physician is the confidence to make quick decisions with limited time, information, and resources. No amount of training or knowledge can supplant low confidence, and patients can sense it immediately.

I remember as a young attending I could sense decreasing confidence in some of the older attendings with whom I worked. They shied away from some of the more complicated cases, and we younger attendings would happily take these more challenging cases. I remember thinking to myself back then, "I hope I never lose my confidence." And yet here I was, starting to feel it—and I couldn't understand why.

To my colleagues and bosses, my performance was great. I was seeing patients quickly, providing great medical care, and achieving high patient-satisfaction results. I posted some of the best numbers in my practice for quite a few years, but I felt increasingly unsure of myself. In fact, one of my older colleagues joked to me privately that emergency medicine is the only profession in which you can become more unsure the more you practice it. Not only do ER physicians rank amongst the highest lawsuit rates of all specialties, but they also deal with the unintended complications of medical procedures from every other specialty. This means that the more an emergency medicine doctor practices, the more acutely she experiences all the different tragic ways the SBIC can fail. We learn quickly, from seeing tens of thousands of cases of our own and our colleagues, that no matter how good a doctor you are, you are going to miss certain things, you are going to make mistakes, and certain things are going to happen to your patients that nobody could predict or prevent.

But we also learn that society is not okay with that. Society wants somebody to blame. Family members want somebody to blame. Hospitals want somebody to blame. Society expects perfection. Doctors aren't supposed to make mistakes. I told my colleagues that being a doctor is like being a wildebeest crossing the Mara River: eventually the crocodile is going to snatch one of us and eat him. And then he'll get another, and another, whenever he so chooses, each and every time a devastating shock to the chosen wildebeest and those around him.

In the ensuing few years I saw some of my colleagues get taken down by crocodile lawsuits while I continued to deal with my own. All the while, Medicare ramped up its "value-based" programs, increasing the documentation burden on physicians and hospitals. During the same period, the first and second generations of electronic medical records (EMR) systems were deployed in hospitals. Although intended to streamline medical documentation, EMRs dramatically reduced physician productivity. This was primarily because the EMR companies got away with designing software with horrendous user interfaces and user workflows. How? Unlike most consumer software, in the sickness-billing world those responsible for purchasing software (the hospital C-suite) are not its end users (the medical staff). The

EMR developers sold the C-suite on "integration," but nobody paid any attention to usability.

And the cost of these systems is astronomical. In May 2018, the Mayo Clinic announced that they were paying $1.5 billion to switch to the Epic EMR system. Pause for a moment: how could software cost $1.5 billion? Well, when your user interface is so unintuitive that you have to hire and deploy an army of consultants and trainers to hold each user's hand for two weeks, it can lead to truly "epic" implementation costs. As if this were not bad enough, the internet buzzed with stories of Epic bullying anybody who criticized its software. Can you imagine the backlash if Microsoft or Google tried to place gag orders to prevent criticism of their software? Yet this is the world of the SBIC. The negative effects of poorly designed EMRs on physician morale and productivity are well documented.

With reimbursement declining due to Medicare's new rules and doctors becoming less productive because of EMRs, physician practices were forced to make their doctors work faster and leaner than ever before.

My experience as a doctor transformed dramatically as a result of all of these changes. With reimbursement going down due to Medicare's new rules and doctors becoming less productive because of EMRs, physician practices expected their doctors to work faster and leaner than ever before. Hospitals expected increasingly higher patient-satisfaction results. Patients and families expected perfection in care and no complications or unexpected events. Insurance companies expected perfectly documented charts, or else no payment. And EMR vendors expected you to use their dreadful software and keep your mouth shut.

These, then, were our directives: Work faster, make everybody happier, document more, and, oh yeah, don't ever make a mistake.

For myself and many of my colleagues, our mindset before beginning an ER shift flipped from eagerness and energetic anticipation to nausea and dread. One of my colleagues developed this dread of ER shifts before even graduating from residency, and promptly quit emergency medicine the day he graduated. Only later did I truly appreciate what he must have felt.

All physicians and nurses, and especially those in our nation's ERs, make personal sacrifices to enter a profession that provides the opportunity and the honor to heal, comfort, and advise their fellow human beings at all hours of the day. They work weekends, overnights, and holidays while most people are sleeping or spending quality time with friends and family. However, when the constituent forces in the SBIC described above repeatedly insult and interfere with the humanity and virtue of medical providers, they do great damage to the provider's ability to empathize.

This loss of empathy is the sickness within our providers to which I referred at the beginning of this essay. Every condition needs a name, so I shall coin the term "empathitis." Empathy, in my personal perspective of its application to the medical profession, is the ability to preserve your sense that you are treating another human being. They're not just "room 12," or "the hypertensive stroke patient," but a human being with a name, a story, family, friends, hopes, and fears—a human being who deserves your full attention, your touch, and your diligent and meticulous thoughtfulness.

Empathitis: an acute or chronic reduction in a person's ability to empathize, often affecting his/her work and life performance.

When the forces surrounding me made it difficult for me to be the type of physician I wanted to be and had trained to be, when those forces repeatedly directed my attention to documentation, billing, EMRs, and moving patients as fast as possible, and when those forces continually chipped away at my mountain of empathy, reducing it to scarcely a handful, I knew the time had come to say goodbye to emergency medicine. My last ER shift was in the summer of 2017.

Luckily, my departure did not signify the end of my medical career. I was fortunate to have worked for a medical practice that gave me the opportunity to develop skills and experience in healthcare technology, data analytics, business development, and telemedicine, and now I have the great pleasure of practicing telemedicine with CirrusMD, an innovative group of amazing human beings who are transforming how healthcare is delivered.

Now, when I see patients from my computer screen, I can chat with them as long as I want. They share stories with me and sometimes we laugh. I advise them the same as I would advise my own family. We don't rush anything. More often than not, they just need reassurance and a little bit of guidance. Although I am no longer placing central lines or doing intubations, I feel more like a true physician than ever before. I spend time talking to patients about health and not just sickness. In addition to dealing with whatever the patient's acute medical condition might be, we talk about food choices, exercise regimens, sleeping habits, behavior modifications, and stress-reduction techniques, and how these things may be connected to the patient's acute condition. Sometimes we discuss fears and anxieties; I've even coached patients through full-blown panic attacks. Now I can truly focus on health and care, not just sickness and billing. Now I operate in a system that I actually like to use and supports me and my mission.

I feel blessed, but I know that many of my former colleagues and friends in the world of emergency medicine continue to endure and suffer. Less than half of my residency class is still practicing traditional emergency medicine. In an era of doctor shortages and long wait times in ERs, I felt this story was important to share, so that you might have some sense as to what lies behind the waiting room door.

Alex Mohseni is a physician innovator and problem solver who is deeply interested in building systems to solve health care's many challenges.

AMAZON, BERKSHIRE HATHAWAY AND JP MORGAN CHASE CAN TO LEAD EMPLOYER SOLUTION TO OPIOID CRISIS ON THE JOURNEY TO LARGER HEALTH CARE REINVENTION

Amazon has proven again and again that Bezos and team can bring fundamental change to multiple industries as he famously said, "Your margin is my opportunity." Adding one of the world's most respected and trusted business figures in Warren Buffett and the leader of one of the largest financial institutions who led it through the 2008 financial crisis in Jamie Dimon and health care's long overdue overhaul may be upon us. [We'll call the partnership ABJ for short.] Not since I wrote Health Insurance's "Bunker Buster"[186] nearly eight years ago have I seen anything that has the potential to bring a brighter future for all Americans if they make the right moves.

With the urgency of solving the opioid crisis, ABJ leadership is needed more than ever. It's clear that the opioid crisis is a unique public health crisis that is also a microcosm of the even larger health care problem. Unlike other public health crises, it's impossible to solve the opioid crisis without significant involvement by employers who are both victims of the crisis and unwitting enablers. As outlined in the rest of the book, the opioid crisis is a systemic and logical outgrowth of a fundamentally flawed model that ABJ can play a catalyzing role in remaking.

Shortly after the initial announcement of the three companies collaborating, I outlined the "10 Mistakes Amazon, Berkshire Hathaway and J.P. Morgan Must Avoid to Make a Dent in Health care.[187] Even though any set of major employers could do many of the things outlined here, conventional employer-led efforts have failed to change health care. Few would call Bezos, Buffett, or Dimon conventional thinkers.

I will spell out below how ABJ could tackle the health care tapeworm (Warren Buffett's term for the negative impact of health care on the U.S. economy). Three key facts potentially differentiate the ABJ health initiative from past employer-led efforts:

1. The strategic focus and attention of three of the most successful CEOs in U.S. history.
2. Warren Buffett's moral authority and trust will give the initiative a bully pulpit that can reach the general public.
3. Amazon and J.P. Morgan Chase's technology, financial structuring, and data prowess can be applied to root out fraud, waste and abuse, create new care pathways, and new revenue and financing models.

If ABJ applies the same discipline to health care that they apply to every other area impacting their business, they can be a model for other employers. Below are ten ways the ABJ initiative could catalyze change in the U.S. health care system with a more detailed explanation below. These won't all necessarily happen but with each item, the likelihood of wholesale transformation increases exponentially.

1. New industry norms for benefits purchasing transparency and conflicts disclosure
2. Cybercrime fraud rates will drop dramatically
3. Fraud awareness will trigger landscape-changing litigation

4. Health care will stop stealing from retirement savings and millennials future
5. Market clarity that employers are the real "insurance" companies
6. Create a spotlight on high rates of overtreatment and misdiagnosis
7. Open source will come to health care
8. Massive new capital restructuring opportunities
9. Primary care rebirth
10. Focus on going local to go national

Now that you know where we're going, let's dive into each point.

1. New industry norms for benefits purchasing transparency and conflicts disclosure

The ABJ leaders each have deep financial services expertise where meaningful disclosure of compensation and conflicts of interest is deeply embedded both legally and culturally. As they dig in, I would expect the ABJ partnership to conclude that new norms in health benefits are needed in this arena, such as what we've developed for the Health Rosetta plan sponsor bill of rights, benefits advisor code of conduct and disclosure standards. These are "motherhood and apple pie" concepts, however they are the polar opposite from current industry norms where benefits brokers frequently sit on both sides of transactions with significant undisclosed conflicts. In particular, bringing transparency to the money flows related to the opioid supply chain is vital to understanding the economic motivation that fueled key players in the benefits supply chain to turn a blind eye to extraordinary rates of opioid prescriptions. The National Safety Council survey showed 99% of doctors are prescribing highly addictive opioid medicines for longer than the three-day period recommended by the Centers for Disease Control and Prevention (CDC).[188] Underlying this data are perverse incentives baked into health plans where non-evidence-based opioid prescriptions are paid for while evidence-based interventions such as PT are either not paid for or are extremely cumbersome to access.

2. Cybercrime fraud rates will drop dramatically

The same sort of algorithms that identify fraud in credit cards can be applied to health care but haven't. Simple to detect fraud like a single claim being paid 25 times to cybercriminals (a real and all-too-common occurrence modern payment integrity services find) are more common than most can imagine. ABJ will also see that blatant fraud is just the tip of the fraud, waste and abuse iceberg. Governor Tommy Thompson is the Chairman of the Board of 4C Health Solutions, a leading payment integrity service provider, who has stated that their software regularly detects claims from suspended doctors prescribing opioids and many other anomalies related to opioid claims. The lack of scrutiny by legacy health claims processors will become self-evident. As outlined in Chapter 10, rates of fraud in health care are where they were in credit cards 20+ years ago when they were over 10%. Today they are well under 1%. It's time for that improvement in health care.

3. Fraud awareness will trigger landscape-changing litigation

Even though cybercrime is the tip of the iceberg on fraud, waste and abuse, it is so blatant that it is already spurring legal activity. In Chapter 26, I quote a Big Four risk management practice leader who said, "ERISA Fiduciary Risk is the Largest Undisclosed Risk I've Seen in my Career." Shareholder fiduciary duty is also snapping large company CEOs to attention as they get awakened to the risk. Activist shareholders are realizing how straightforward it is to improve earnings by slaying the health care cost beast.

For example, a multinational manufacturer implemented a proper musculoskeletal management program by having physical therapists working with employees and workplace ergonomics. Even with just 35% of the targeted employees getting into the program, that had an overall 1.7% positive impact on company earnings. At a human level, mismanagement of musculoskeletal issues is one of the big on-ramps to opioid misuse. For example, there are tremendous volumes of non-evidence-based opioid prescriptions for lower back pain as well as non-evidence-based spinal procedures that are followed by opioid prescriptions.

4. Health care will stop stealing from retirement savings, millennials future and small businesses

Health care has crushed the average boomer's retirement savings by $1 million.[189] Even if this estimate is off by 10x (unlikely), it's still $7.6 trillion that could have been under management by financial firms such as JP Morgan. My senior level contacts in the 401k/retirement segment surprised me when they said that government de-privatizing of retirement (due to low savings levels) is on the worry list of folks such as Jamie Dimon. If true, it is another reason organizations like JP Morgan Chase would want to redirect money being squandered in health care to retirement accounts.

As outlined in Chapter 6, health care is on track to consume half of a typical millennial's lifetime earnings. As the largest generation in history and entering the age when that consumer purchasing and retirement savings are greatest, millennials are the most important generation for all of the ABJ organizations. Smart employers also find they are natural early adopters of Health Rosetta type benefits programs that spread to the rest of the employees.

Perhaps the most underestimated opportunity available to ABJ are the customers and partners of ABJ businesses. Amazon Marketplace and JP Morgan Chase's retail banks have millions of business customers. They can use their communication channels to educate their customers and partners. Money squandered in health care holds back commerce and deposits that each of those organizations could be facilitating.

5. Market clarity that employers are the real "insurance" companies

Employers realizing they are, in fact, carrying the financial risk of health insurance is the health plan industry's worst nightmare.[190] There is a growing realization that since less than a third of the claims insurance companies process actually put the insurance companies' money at risk, "insurance" companies are more appropriately described as commoditize-able claims processors. It is self-evident that paying a third-party to manage risk when they benefit from *rising* costs hasn't worked out well. The smart health insurance companies already understand this and their investments demonstrate they already have come to this conclusion – each has been aggressively diversifying out of the insurance business. They are happy to milk the insurance business until it goes away but, their corporate development actions clearly signal what they believe their future is. For example, I heard Aetna CEO, Mark Bertolini, say at a Health 2.0 conference that Aetna increasingly sees themselves as a technology company with insurance on the side. [See Chapter 5, *What You Don't Know About the Pressures and Constraints Facing Insurance Executives Costs You Dearly* for a deeper explanation.]

For all but health care, insurance is used for unforeseen risks. Much of what is spent on health "insurance" is more akin to pre-paid and/or budgeted health care for things that are entirely predictable year over year whether it's flu season or a number of common procedures such as surgeries. The *real* insurance is stop-loss insurance sometimes called reinsurance. Berkshire happens to be one of the top reinsurance firms in the world. The few times that the firms we think of as health insurance companies took on risk was with the ACA exchanges. Their inability to manage risk was demonstrated as they floundered around for a few years before making money and the result was a dramatic spike in rates. In contrast, Berkshire brings decades of experience managing highly unpredictable risk. As outlined in Chapters 5 and 18, forward-looking mayors already see a critical need with 35% of the workforce having no employer-provided health benefits. Considering that 94% of all job growth was in these areas, it's not hard to see why this is on their mind. It's not hard to imagine city and county-based health insurance cooperatives controlled by their local community that is reinsured by Berkshire. It would be a public-private partnership that is the rough equivalent of the Medicaid buy-in efforts that have gained traction in states such as Nevada that would make competitively priced health benefits that isn't tied to a specific employer – an artifact of World War II that Dr. Gawande pointed out in his first interview following his CEO announcement.

6. Create a spotlight on high rates of overtreatment and misdiagnosis

ABJ's leadership will see studies such as the Starbucks/Virginia Mason study that found 90% of spinal procedures did not help at all. The new ABJ CEO, Dr. Atul Gawande, is well aware of the extraordinary rates of misdiagnosis across health care, like what I outline in Chapter 14, *Centers of Excellence Offer a Golden Opportunity*. Naturally, they want to ensure their employees get the best possible care, which also saves tremendous money. It's commonly known that 30-50% of what we do to people in health care does not make them better and could make them worse. One of the foremost experts in employer benefits, Brian Klepper, estimates that 2% of the entire U.S. economy is tied up in non-evidence-based, non-value-add musculoskeletal procedures.

7. Open source will come to health care

As much as companies such as Amazon keep some information and code proprietary, they also actively benefit from open source. Open source software underpins major parts of Amazon's business. Some problems are too big to tackle on your own. As big as ABJ is, they aren't big enough to tackle all of health care and they don't have dominant market share in any single geography. Because adoption happens so slowly in health care, Health Rosetta is catalyzing the creation of a Wikipedia-like resource for the next 50 years of health (a group of visionary doctors call their vision Health 3.0) is to dramatically accelerate the rate of adoption for successful approaches. Those insights will benefit ABJ.

In the other direction, ABJ should be motivated to share what they are doing with other local employers to more rapidly change norms in a given health care market. ABJ, alone, isn't big enough to transform a local health care market without an alliance with other employers. While the Fair Trade-like model for health care outlined in Chapter 11 is non-controversial outside of health care, ABJ can add heft and use their bully pulpit to normalize more appropriate behavior in this area. For example, legitimate pricing[191] versus the arguably predatory and arbitrary pricing today would still let health care providers to set their prices (i.e., not government set) but it would be consistent and known across all health care purchasers. One Health Rosetta component— Transparent Open Networks (see Chapter 22) —already enables this. In other words, health care transactions could operate like every other part of the economy. **Single pricing is a subtle, but critical, part of making health care functional.** *Not* **tackling this would be one of the biggest mistakes ABJ could make.** Practically speaking, this can be done locale by locale unless the federal government completely took over pricing for the country.

Unlike past failed employer-led efforts, ABJ have a tremendous number of small business customers/partners. If ABJ plays its cards right, the least interesting facet of their alliance are their 1 million+ employees as they touch far more through the reach of their business. One way of looking at this is the best way for them to get the most financial gain in the long-term is to avoid the short-sighted, parochial approaches of past employer-led efforts that kept all the gains for themselves. Over time, provider organizations were adept at dividing and conquering and nothing fundamentally changed. Instead, ABJ can invite any willing business to participate on both the demand and supply side of the health care equation into a fair marketplace.

8. Massive new capital restructuring opportunities

This item could be an entire white paper, but I'll touch on just two opportunities stemming from the above items. Hundreds of billions of dollars (if not more) have been and are being tied up in fraud, waste and abuse. As large purchasers and others begin to account for this, a subset of it can be treated as bad debt and turned into financial instruments that are sold to opportunistic, sophisticated investors. The subsequent collection efforts by these purchasers would be dramatic to any person or organization enabling the fraud. Second, it is well known that we have at least 40% over-capacity of hospital beds, fueled by a massive revenue bond bubble. The orderly disposition and restructuring of these assets is another massive opportunity that can be accelerated by the work of ABJ and others. Outside of rural settings that have fewer over-capacity issues, evidence shows that hospital closings have no impact on outcomes.[192]

9. Primary care rebirth

Just based on the number of employees ABJ has, it makes economic sense to fund ~1500 value-based primary care clinics. They can de-risk this investment by making it available to ABJ partners and business and retail customers. Once again, it's enlightened self-interest to open these clinics to anyone in their communities starting with their own employees, then their customers' employees and ultimately to anyone. ABJ can dramatically reduce their investment simply by plugging into existing value-based primary care practices such as independent direct primary care practices that are open to being paid directly by employers. I wasn't surprised that ABJ recently hired my parent's primary care physician who has deep experience in a vanguard value-based primary care organization. As outlined throughout the book, solving the opioid crisis and the larger health care problem is impossible without rebuilding the devastated primary care system in this country that has led to so many problems. [See Chapter 21 for more on value-based primary care.]

10. Focus on going local to go national

From Facebook to Thumbtack to Uber/Lyft, the best way to go national with something game-changing is to start with a hyperlocal focus. This lets you prove unit economics in a controllable environment. I often draw an analogy between the Health

Rosetta and LEED for many reasons. One of them is that certain locales were early adopters of LEED before it spread nationwide and the same is happening with the Health Rosetta.

For example, Portland, Oregon was an early adopter of LEED and it has grown a cluster of sustainable industries by attracting talent and businesses to the area. Over the last year, I have been gathering feedback on creating a competition like Google Fiber or Amazon HQ2 competitions to identify communities where the new health ecosystem forms. ABJ could collaborate on this, if desired.

Beyond the obvious benefits of defining and pioneering the next century of health, solving the opioid crisis is a profound imperative. As I pointed out in Chapter 1: *The Opioid Crisis Isn't an Anomaly*, the largest public health crisis in 100 years has major employer/economic implications and is simply impossible to solve without active employer involvement. The sad fact is that every addict needs an enabler and employers have been the biggest (unwitting) enabler for 11 of the 12 major drivers of the crisis. The silver lining is that solving the opioid crisis takes you a long way towards solving broader health care dysfunction. Employers implementing Health Rosetta type benefits have much lower rates of opioid use disorders due to the upstream "antidotes" to the crisis such as greatly improved primary care and avoidance of non-evidence-based approaches to musculoskeletal issues.

In short, ABJ has the power to demonstrate that employer health benefits are the newspaper classifieds of transforming the health care business

Health care has many analogies with another industry that has been dominated by regional monopolies/oligopolies—newspapers. Like employer health benefits, the classifieds business was very easy to overlook. However, in both cases, they drove a significant majority of profits for newspapers. Once the classifieds business was impacted by the Internet, the newspaper industry was never the same. If the ABJ initiative plays its cards right, they can catalyze restoring the American Dream for millions of Americans by fixing health care. The great news is that there are many microcosms in the U.S. where the best health care system in the world exists — far more affordable and effective than we're used to. ABJ has the opportunity to help America leapfrog the rest of the world and finally have a truly superior and efficient health care system.

DECODING A FULLY INSURED RENEWAL

Wes Spencer

A health insurance renewal is not as complicated as it seems. Although you may be unfamiliar with the terminology used in renewal documentation, each section and calculation is intended to predict a premium that (when paid) will fund the following:

BUCKET 1: Upcoming 12 months medical & Rx claims (what we want paid).
BUCKET 2: Stop-Loss premiums to reduce exposure to high cost claimants.
BUCKET 3: Carrier's operating expenses & profit (negotiable).

The following is an actual de-identified 2018 renewal; yours will look similar:

Renewal Development - Detailed Projections

	Medical	Prescription Drug	Dental	Vision	Total
Average Monthly Employees Enrolled in Experience Period	163	163			163
Average Monthly Members Enrolled in Experience Period	341	341			341
1. Approved Charges	$1,819,597	$531,207			$2,350,804
Less : Provider Reimbursement Savings	$887,609	$264,249			$1,151,858
Less : Member Liability	$248,556	$37,710			$286,266
2. Claims Paid in Experience Period	$683,432	$228,880			$912,312
Less : Large Claim Payment	$130,253	$3,216			$133,469
3. Net Claims Considered for Rating Projection	$553,179	$225,664			$778,843
Plus : Estimate Incurred But Not Reported Claims	$32,648	$384			$33,032
4. Total Incurred Claims	$585,827	$226,048			$811,875
Annualized Incurred Claims	$585,827	$226,048			$811,875
5. Adjustment for Membership and Benefit Changes during the experience period	$49,316	($8,350)			$40,966
Annualized Incurred Claims adjusted for benefit and membership changes	$635,143	$217,698			$852,840
Effective Trend	1.0818	1.1965			1.1111
6. Trended Claims	$687,111	$260,484			$947,595
Plus : Estimate Provider Adjustment	$48,892	($44,543)			$4,350
Plus : Large Claims up to Attachment Point	$97,591	$2,409			$100,000
Plus : Capitation	$62,527	$0			$62,527
Plus : Adjustment for Credibility	($30,735)	$568			($30,167)
7. Projected Claims for the Rating Period	$865,863	$218,919			$1,084,305
Plus : Pooling Charges	$146,758	$24,790			$171,548
Plus : Projected Retention Expenses	$256,268	$29,876			$286,144
Less : Cap/Floor Adjustment	$0	$0			$0
8. Projected Total Expenses for the Rating Period	$1,268,413	$273,585			$1,541,998
9. Projected Income Required for the Rating Period	$1,268,413	$273,585			$1,541,998
10. Annual Income at Current Rates	$1,123,983	$241,059			$1,365,043
11. Change in Rates for the Rating Period expressed as a Percentage Change from your Current Rates	12.85%	13.49%			12.96%

Some variances may occur to rounding

Experience Period : (Incurred: 08/2016-07/2017), (Paid: 08/2016-08/2017)

Here's how it looks when we categorize into the three "buckets":

Renewal Development - Detailed Projections

	Medical	Prescription Drug	Dental	Vision	Total
Average Monthly Employees Enrolled in Experience Period	163	163			163
Average Monthly Members Enrolled in Experience Period	341	341			341
1. Approved Charges	$1,819,597	$531,207			$2,350,804
Less : Provider Reimbursement Savings	$887,609	$264,249			$1,151,858
Less : Member Liability	$248,556	$37,710	Claims - Medical & Rx		$286,266
2. Claims Paid in Experience Period	$683,432	$228,880	$1,270,988 Total Claims		$912,312
Less : Large Claim Payment	$130,253	$3,216	$286,266 Members		$133,469
3. Net Claims Considered for Rating Projection	$553,179	$225,664			$778,843
Plus : Estimate Incurred But Not Reported Claims	$32,648	$384	$984,402 Claims Paid		$33,032
4. Total Incurred Claims	$585,827	$226,048			$811,875
Annualized Incurred Claims	$585,827	$226,048	Stop Loss Insurance		$811,875
5. Adjustment for Membership and Benefit Changes during the experience period	$49,316	($8,350)	$171,548		$40,966
Annualized Incurred Claims adjusted for benefit and membership changes	$635,143	$217,698	($73,460) Paid Over spec.		$852,840
Effective Trend	1.0818	1.1965			1.1111
6. Trended Claims	$687,111	$260,484	$138,079 Profit		$947,595
Plus : Estimate Provider Adjustment	$48,892	($44,543)			$4,350
Plus : Large Claims up to Attachment Point	$97,591	$2,409	Operations & Profit		$100,000
Plus : Capitation	$62,527	$0	$94,750 Trend		$62,527
Plus : Adjustment for Credibility	($30,735)	$568	$4,350 Provider Adj. $286,144 Retention		($30,167)
7. Projected Claims for the Rating Period	$865,863	$218,919	($30,167) Credibility		$1,084,305
Plus : Pooling Charges	$146,758	$24,790	$138,079 Stop Loss Prft.		$171,548
Plus : Projected Retention Expenses	$256,268	$29,876	$493,156 (50% claims)		$286,144
Less : Cap/Floor Adjustment	$0	$0	$3,025 PEPY		$0
8. Projected Total Expenses for the Rating Period	$1,268,413	$273,585	$252.12 PEPM		$1,541,998
9. Projected Income Required for the Rating Period	$1,268,413	$273,585			$1,541,998
10. Annual Income at Current Rates	$1,123,983	$241,059			$1,365,043
11. Change in Rates for the Rating Period expressed as a Percentage Change from your Current Rates	12.85%	13.49%			12.96%

Some variances may occur to rounding

Experience Period : (Incurred: 08/2016-07/2017), (Paid: 08/2016-08/2017)

BUCKET 1. Upcoming 12 months medical & Rx claims.

The important facts to consider are included below. I have omitted "Provider Reimbursement Savings" as this is simply a way of marketing a discount that is superficial at best. This discount is the amount purportedly negotiated from the Approved Charges submitted by providers. The Approved Charges come from the provider/hospital "Charge Master", which is grossly inflated to account for the agreed discount. We need to focus on what is actually paid. Here's how to add it all up:

Net Claims Considered for Rating Projection $778,843

This number is derived by taking Approved Charges, deducting discounts (above), member liability (deductibles, coinsurance, & copays), and removing "high claimant" charges. This is where we start.

Add: IBNR (Incurred but not received) $33,032

IBNR is a legitimate consideration due to claim billing lag. However, this amount only represents an estimate.

Add: Large Claims Up to Attachment Point $100,000

Although this is in the "Trended Claims" section of the report, include this in your total claim calculations. In this example it is $100,000, which represents the amount paid for a high claimant. Yes, it looks like self-insuring and it is, in a way. The difference is that you pay for it about one year after it is incurred (at your renewal). So, in this example, the group had only one employee exceed the "pooling point" or "attachment point." Thus, $100,000 is added back. We'll discuss this further in Stop-Loss below.

Add: Capitation $62,527

This may be a new term for you, but it's actually pretty simple. Instead of the carrier paying primary care providers per visit, they pay selected in-network PCPs a fixed monthly amount for each of your members who nominate a "capitated provider." This amount is paid whether or not your employee goes to the doctor. If your employee does not have a regular doctor, a capitated provider is assigned. In this case, it equates to $183.36 per member (including spouses and children). This pays for about two visits per year. You may pay more for capitation, and I believe it discourages quality care. Here are a few important questions to consider:

Do you think every member goes to the PCP two times a year?

If the PCP cannot bill insurance for your visit, are they motivated to spend time with you?
If you're on an HSA plan, does the member still pay for the visit, even if your PCP is "capitated?"
Is the HMO network restrictive enough to steer patients to low cost, high quality providers?

TOTAL Claims Paid: $984,402 [not listed]

This amount is not specifically listed on the renewal example above. However, it is the most important statistic you need to calculate (see the green bubble). It includes all Medical & Rx incurred for a 12-month period.

BUCKET 2. Stop-Loss premiums to reduce exposure to high cost claimants.

You may be aware of the reinsurance market if you've ever considered self-funding. Primarily known as stop-loss insurance, it is purchased by fully-insured carriers and self-funded employers alike.

Pooling Charges: $171,546

This amount is the cost of stop-loss insurance for severe, high cost claims. It is the premium you pay for the insurance company to accept this risk. In this example, your responsibility is the first $100,000 of a big claim. Called the "attachment point" or pooling point, payments in excess of $100,000 per member, are excluded from your claim experience & premium calculation. (NOTE: I've seen this credit conveniently omitted, make sure you see it in writing). The $100,000 deductible includes medical and Rx payments combined, per member. So, if you have 10 members exceed $100,000, your renewal will reflect a $1,000,000 increase, plus everything else!

Less: Large Claim Payments: $133,469, but really only $33,469....

In section 2 [Less large claims payments], you see $133,469 was removed from "Claims Paid in Experience Period" (This is the credit you're looking for). This means that the entire group of large claimants had a total of $133,469 in claims paid. In section 6 [Large Claim Payments up to Attachment Point] you see $100,000 added back to your premium calculation. This tells you two things; there was only one large claimant, and the stop-loss insurance paid a net $33,469 after receiving $171,546 in premium.

BUCKET 3. Carrier operating expenses & profit.

One question to ask as we review each of these "buckets" is: if my group maintains historical medical utilization, who keeps the proceeds from each bucket? When you're negotiating a fully-insured renewal, every dollar increase is spread over your monthly single/double/family rate for 12 months.

Adjustment for Membership & Benefit Changes, ADD: $40,966

Adjustments will be applied for group demographic changes. Demographic changes include high turnover, mid-year open enrollment that changes member responsibility, or a group wide benefit change. In this example, the group chose to add a 5th tier to the Rx card, resulting in a higher copay for members taking specialty drugs. This should reduce premium. However, high turnover is also present in this group. Ask for clarity on what changed and why any adjustments were made that increased the premium.

Effective Trend: 1.1111 or ADD: $94,755.

Actuarially, trend is the year-over-year % increase in claims expense. Practically, it is a function that insurance companies and health care providers use to automatically increase revenue. Trend is a historical look back that is then projected forward. This creates a self-fulfilling prophecy, resulting in an auto-increase for both your insurance company, and the health care providers they pay. It has been accepted as norm for years. Fight the urge to accept this as fact.

Previously, I mentioned if you're considering self-funding, you should apply a "trend" factor to your Expected Claims budget. I only recommend this if you have poor claims data. It's your money to budget and if trend is less than expected, you win. Good carriers have nearly perfect claims data, and projected claims in excess of your current claims period should only be justified by knowledge of an ongoing/new high claimant(s).

Don't let carriers automatically apply trend to your premium. Instead, ask them to provide the last two year's contract with the hospitals in your area showing the charge master and discount per CPT code. Also, ask for your PBM's (prescription benefit manager) prescription contract with retail cost of each drug and the carrier's own discounted rate. If trend is in excess of Consumer Price Index (CPI normally about 2%), ask why the cost was allowed to increase.

Estimated Provider Adjustments, ADD: $4,350

This is, again, a fairly opaque adjustment. When I asked what this adjustment includes, here is the response from the carrier: "Benefit expense items that do not run through our claims processing systems. These items include payments to providers for risk arrangements, hospital settlements, provider incentives and pharmacy rebates."

If we break that down, essentially, it's a bucket of adjustments for paying or receiving money outside of contract. For example, drug manufacturers provide rebates as a result of PBM negotiation. Depending on your PBM, you receive 0-100% of these rebates as credit towards your renewal. In our example, one can assume that the carrier received $44,543 in Rx rebates.

However, this was "washed out" by $48,892 in risk arrangements, hospital settlements, or provider incentives. Ask for details on these expenses that apply directly to your group. Specifically, get the list of Rx rebates received showing total rebate, carrier retention, and your credit. As for risk arrangements and hospital settlements, if it doesn't apply directly to your group, ask for it to be removed.

ADD: Projected Retention Expense, ADD: $286,144

This is a clever way to say "markup." Here is the carrier's actual definition:

"The amount charged to customers to cover the costs of providing services. This includes: claim processing, customer service, wellness and care management, access to carrier negotiated provider discounts and data and analytics (reporting)."

Don't get me wrong, markup is necessary to cover operations, G&A, overhead, and profit. Without markup, we cannot operate. So, the best way to analyze this line item is to benchmark against industry peers. In this example, the $286,144 represents this carrier's markup. However, to make this number meaningful, we need to change it to a PEPM (per employee per month) cost. This group has 163 enrolled, so the PEPM is $146.29, with a member/employee ratio of 2.09.

Below are some recent industry-peer mark-ups. I've included claim processing, customer service, wellness & care management, network negotiation fees, claims reporting, and agent commission in each of these benchmarks:

-Carrier #1: $146.29 PEPM (fully-insured) & $96.65 PEPM (self-funded)
-Carrier #2: $85.55 PEPM (fully-insured) & $78.56 PEPM (self-funded)
-Carrier #3: $69.10 PEPM (self-funded)
-Carrier #4: $52.49 PEPM + hourly case management (self-funded)
-Clearly, Carrier #1 is nearly 3x the lowest competitor in the market, and represents the highest markup.

Accordingly, one would expect a significant benefit for this markup. To validate this, ask the following simple questions:

-Are you receiving claims processing worth 200%-300% of market?
-Are you receiving customer service worth 200-300% of market?
-Are you receiving wellness & care management worth 200-300% of market?
-If I'm paying 11% trend, is the network negotiation worth 200-300% of market?
-Is claims transparency, analytics, and plan counseling worth 200-300% of market?
-Is my agent/advisor receiving 200-300% ofmarket commission to service my account?

CONCLUSION

Hopefully, this helps sheds light on the way an insurance carrier calculates a renewal premium, so you have leverage at the negotiating table. In this example, $493,156 (50% markup on claims) could flow through to the insurance carrier.

That's $3,025 per enrolled employee per year! What would that mean to your bottom line and/or employees' wallet?

BENEFITS OPTIONS FOR SMALL BUSINESSES AND SOLE PROPRIETORS

By David Contorno

I am a small business (or individual)… how can I create a benefits package in the Health Rosetta mindset?

Health Rosetta is more a mindset than a single strategy, a collection of principles and practices rather than a health plan. While there are some regulatory and market conditions that make it easier to follow this model as an employer group gets larger, there are still some things that anyone can do.

Small Businesses

Within the ACA, a small employer was defined as one with fewer than 100 full time equivalent employees (FTEs). However, in October 2015, President Obama signed the PACE act allowing each state to decide to either keep its traditional definition (50 employees in most cases) or go to 100. Most states opted to keep it at 50, although some states, NY for example, moved it or kept it at 100. So, from a regulatory perspective, 50 employees or fewer seems to be the most common "small group." As an employer moves up in size, some of the financing side strategies definitely become easier.

Although all of our strategies are common sense, they are still innovative to health care, and small businesses do have to get even more "non-traditional" to accomplish similar results. The primary reason is that the ACA put more restrictions on the products insurance carriers can offer in this space; in addition, there is the possibility that larger-sized small employers may be subject to certain ACA mandates that these plans may not comply with.

Mandates, however, do not apply to most employers under 50 FTEs. This means there is no penalty for offering non-ACA compliant plans (or even no coverage). For this size employer, there are a few potential solutions:

1. Contract with a local direct primary care (DPC) doctor for your employees. Studies show that for about 80 percent of people, a proper functioning primary care home can provide 100 percent of the care they need. The national average cost is $50-$150 per employee per month. There are generally no additional fees, no co-pays, and no claims to file.
2. Primary care alone cannot serve the needs of the remaining 20 percent and can leave other people anxious about the "what if's". In this case, a "health sharing plan" can provide that additional protection. While many of these plans came out of a faith-based exemption under the ACA, several have developed in recent years that either remove or significantly downplay the religious affiliation requirements. Ironically, although most sharing organizations want to avoid any traditional insurance terms, for fear of being regulated like insurance, most operate the way insurance was always intended to operate: All members pay enough into the pot to fund judicious and fair disbursements of benefits to cover moderate to large medical encounters. (The small to moderate stuff should either be paid for out of pocket or handled by the DPC doctor mentioned in #1 above.) A good sharing program will recog-

nize the benefits of DPC and give a discount on the membership fees when included. I priced out a family of four, with DPC and the sharing program (with an initial patient responsibility of $1000 per medical need) in Western North Carolina and the total cost for all was well under $700 per month for the whole family. I have seen many single premiums in traditional programs at this price point lately.

3. If DPC is not an option, either because you have a highly distributed workforce or because there simply aren't any near you, you may still be able to bring in many of its benefits of primary care in a virtual format. Generally, this costs around $100 per month for an employee.

4. Lastly, as the Association Health Plan (AHP) Rule rolls out, it *may* offer an opportunity for employers to more easily band together. Contrary to widespread misconceptions, I believe this will only give such groups access to limited benefits. However, it could lift small businesses out of the small group market, which operates under community rating requirements. If so, this would allow a Health Rosetta advisor to construct a plan that truly addresses incentives designed to reward quantity over quality in ways not otherwise available to smaller groups.

Larger Small Businesses

As an employer moves out of the 50-employee market, regulations become more onerous, but at the same time, it becomes easier to operate in a Health Rosetta environment. Here are a few points to consider for employers of 50 to about 100:

1. Contrary to popular belief, self-insured does not inherently mean more risky; it can actually be less risky than a fully insured plan if you want it to be. Risk can be the result of an inexperienced benefits broker but it can also be a deliberate choice. Due to the pressure the ACA applied to fully insured plans, there are today many new forms of protection or risk

management for smaller employers, e.g., aggregate-only policies, spaggregate, monthly aggregate accommodation, non-laserable contracts, and, as mentioned in #2, level funding (not to be confused with carrier-based level funding).

2. Not all self-inured plans are created equal. If you take a fully insured large carrier plan, and put that same plan, PPO network, pharmacy benefit management, etc., into a self-insured model, you have functionally changed absolutely nothing. You still have relinquished full control of both costs and utilization to an entity that benefits as costs rise. Also, most carriers expressly prohibit Health Rosetta principles because they actively lower costs—which in turn lowers their profit.

3. A "level funded plan" is often viewed as a safe, "dip a toe in the water" path to becoming self-insured. When the carriers saw this happening, they came out with their own versions and designed them to maximize profit. They do this by inflating the fixed costs, reducing the claims funding, and, in the rare case where there is leftover claims funding, keeping one-third to one-half of what you overpaid. With a proper level-funded model, the self-insured employer gets far more control, far more flexibility, reduced fixed costs, and 100 percent of the excess claims funding back.

4. Once an employer determines that it can construct a financially feasible self-insured arrangement with a proper third-party administrator and PBM, all the Health Rosetta principles can easily be applied.

5. These plans can and should be designed to meet all the ACA mandates for both the employer and the individual.

Individuals

What can you do as an employee not in a decision-making capacity at a company, or as someone who is self-employed or unemployed? You can do a lot! First off, please remember that health insurance does *not* equal health care. Health insurance is just one way to pay for care. Another is the health sharing programs mentioned above, which have been operating for a couple of decades and are used by approximately one million people.[193] And there is still another way: It's called cash.

The tens of millions of people with high deductible plans can save enormous sums by using cash, as demonstrated by my own hernia operation. Even using a facility 800 miles away from my home, which had much higher quality than any in my area, and paying 100 percent of my own costs, including travel, I paid one-third of what my out-of-pocket would have been had I stayed local and used a traditional insurance plan. Most of the time, you do not need to travel anywhere near that far to find a high-quality facility, but if you were going to get way better care and save thousands of dollars, wouldn't you be willing to?

These same principles can be applied to prescriptions. Especially with generics, the cash price is often below your plan's co-pay. And when you unknowingly overpay for the drug by showing your insurance ID card, you are actually hurting yourself down the road in the form of higher premiums—and you are often hurting the pharmacy thanks to "clawbacks." This is when your plan's PBM pulls back the difference between the co-pay and cost of the drug in order to enhance their profits, even though they literally provided no value, especially in that particular transaction.

It may not be easy, because the system doesn't want it to be, but for an individual, the solution is relatively simple: You need to demand total cost and quality information (getting that is the hard part), compare these data with your insurance coverage, and only then decide where to go for care. Instead, most Americans take an "insurance first" approach. In nearly all other economic transactions, we determine best value first, then we figure out how to get the money needed to pay for it. If we all did that in health care, things would change for the positive *very* rapidly.

AUTHOR BIO

D ave Chase is an industry ecosystem thinker and shifter. He is a founder of Health Rosetta, a blueprint for high-performance health benefits that accelerates adoption of simple, practical, nonpartisan fixes to our health care system and provides certification for benefits professionals (healthrosetta.org). Health Rosetta was formally launched in September 2017 with the release of Chase's last book, *The CEO's Guide to Restoring the American Dream*, which focuses on how high-performing organizations have solved health care's toughest challenges, as does his TEDx talk, "Health Care Stole the American Dream—Here's How We Take It Back." With the publication of *The Opioid Crisis Wake-up Call*, Health Rosetta it is set to move into the next phase, including events, online communities, employer memberships, certifications, local chapters, and enabling technology. In the first year of existence, the program has grown to include benefits advisors whose clients provide health benefits for nearly 5 million Americans.

Chase co-edited the seminal book on patient engagement, *Engage! Transforming Healthcare Through Digital Patient Engagement*, published by HIMSS in 2013, wrote the seminal paper on "Direct Primary Care" and founded the most successful technology platform in health care.

As a leader of the industry association for digital advertising (Interactive Advertising Bureau), Chase also played a driving role in turning the digital advertising market around in the aftermath of the dotcom bust; his work involving research, industry standards, and education programs contributed to it becoming the leading advertising market, surpassing print, broadcast, and cable TV.

Chase has been active in social ventures and is a student of social enterprises and movements that range from the sustainable building industry to microcredit and rural hospital development in the developing world to the remaking of the U.S. food system.

Chase was the CEO and Cofounder of Avado, acquired by and integrated into WebMD and Medscape. Before Avado, Chase spent several years outside of health care in startups as a founder or in consulting roles with LiveRez.com, MarketLeader, and WhatCounts. He was also on the founding and leadership teams in two $1 billion+ businesses within Microsoft, including their $2 billion health care platform business.

Chase is a husband, father of two student athletes, and oxygen-fueled mountain athlete. His team placed 3rd in their division and 24th overall (of 500 teams) in the oldest adventure race in the U.S. where Dave tackled the Nordic ski leg. Dave is also a former PAC-12 800 Meter competitor.

END NOTES

[1] Berardo, Richie. "2017's States with the Best & Worst School Systems," WalletHub, accessed January 14, 2018, https://wallethub.com/edu/states-with-the-best-schools/5335/

[2] Alan R. Weil and Rachel Dolan, "Confronting Our Nation's Opioid Crisis," The Aspen Health Strategy Group, accessed April 25, 2018, https://asset-saspeninstitute.org/content/uploads/2018/01/AHSG-Final-Report-2017_compressed-2.pdf

[3] Kellermann, A. L. and D. I. Auerbach. "Health Care Cost Growth Is Hurting Middle-Class Families," The Rand Blog, accessed January 3, 2018, http://www.rand.org/blog/2013/01/health-care-cost-growth-is-hurting-middle-class-families.html

[4] Kolodny, Andrew et al. "The Prescription Opioid and Heroin Crisis: A Public Health Approach to an Epidemic of Addiction," Annual Review of Public Health, 36(2015): 559, accessed July 4, 2017, doi:10.1146/annurev-publhealth-031914-122957

[5] Frieden, Thomas R., MD, MPH. and Debra Houry, MD, MPH "Reducing the Risks of Relief — The CDC Opioid-Prescribing Guideline," New England Journal of Medicine 374(2016): 1501-1504, accessed July 4, 2017, doi: 10.1056/NEJMp1515917

[6] Chou, Roger, MD et al. "The Effectiveness and Risks of Long-Term Opioid Therapy for Chronic Pain: A Systematic Review for a National Institutes of Health Pathways to Prevention Workshop," Annual Internal Medicine 162 (2015): 4, accessed July 4, 2017, doi: 10.7326/M14-2559

[7] Lembke, Anna, MD; Keith Humphreys, PhD; and Jordan Newmark, MD. "Weighing the Risks and Benefits of Chronic Opioid Therapy," American Family Physician, accessed July 4, 2017 www.aafp.org/afp/2016/0615/p982. html

[8] Fain, Kevin M., JD, MPH and G. Caleb Alexander, MD, MS. "Mind the Gap: Understanding the Effects of Pharmaceutical Direct-to-Consumer Advertising," Medical Care 52(2014): 4, accessed July 4, 2017, doi: 10.1097/ MLR.0000000000000126

[9] Freburger, Janet K., PT, PhD, et al. "Rising Prevalence of Chronic Low Back Pain," Arch Intern Med. 169(2009): 3, accessed July 4, 2017, doi: 10.1001/ archinternmed.2008.543

[10] Monnat, Shannon. "Deaths of Despair and Support for Trump in the 2016 Presidential Election," The Pennsylvania University Department of Agricultural Economics, Sociology, and Education Research Brief, accessed July 4, 2017. http://aese.psu.edu/directory/smm67/Election16.pdf

[11] Hollingsworth, Alex, Christopher J. Ruhm, and Kosali Simon, "Macroeconomic Conditions and Opioid Abuse," The National Bureau of Economic Research, accessed July 4, 2017, http://www.nber.org/papers/w23192

[12] "Bureau of Labor Statistics for 2016," Social Security Administration, accessed October 24, 2017, https://www.ssa.gov/cgi-bin/netcomp.cgi?-year=2016

[13] Rabin, Roni Caryn. "15-Minute Visits Take a Toll on the Doctor-Patient Relationship," accessed December 29, 2017 https://khn.org/news/15-minute-doctor-visits

[14] Viadro, Christopher. "Increase in Opiate Usage Appears Tied to Decrease in Access to Treatment in Worker's Compensation," ButlerViadro, LLP, accessed July 4, 2017, http://www.butlerviadro.com/blog/2016/05/increase-in-opiate-usage-appears-tied-to-decrease-in-access-to-treatment-in-workers-compensation.shtml

[15] Connor, Vickie. "Patients with Mental Disorders Get Half of All Opioid Prescriptions," accessed July 4, 2017, http://khn.org/news/patients-with-mental-disorders-get-half-of-all-opioid-prescriptions/

[16] Fenton, Joshua J. MD, MPH et al. "The Cost of Satisfaction: A National Study of Patient Satisfaction, Health Care Utilization, Expenditures, and Mortality" Arch Intern Med. 172(2012): 5, accessed July 4, 2017, doi: 10.1001/archinternmed.2011.1662

[17] Robbins, Rebecca. "Do Americans Really Watch 16 Hours of Pharma Ads a Year?," STAT News, accessed September 12, 2017, https://www.statnews.com/2017/09/12/americans-16-hours-pharma-ads/

[18] "New Research Reveals the Trends and Risk Factors Behind America's Growing Heroin Epidemic," CDC, accessed July 4, 2017, https://www.cdc.gov/media/releases/2015/p0707-heroin-epidemic.html

[19] Katz, Josh. "Drug Deaths in America Are Rising Faster Than Ever," The New York Times, accessed July 4, 2017, https://www.nytimes.com/interactive/2017/06/05/upshot/opioid-epidemic-drug-overdose-deaths-are-rising-faster-than-ever.html

[20] Cutter, Chip. "The opioid crisis is creating a fresh hell for America's employers," accessed August 4, 2017, https://www.linkedin.com/pulse/opioid-crisis-creating-fresh-hell-americas-employers-chip-cutter/

[21] DeWine, Mike. "Economic Aspects of Opioid Crisis" Filmed June 2017 at Longworth House Office Building, Washington D.C. Video 26:41. https://www.youtube.com/watch?v=LIQIQ1jC2dg&feature=youtu.be&t=1601

[22] Donnelly, Frank. "Staten Island Ferry Ex-Captain Details Chaos That Enveloped Barberi after Fatal Crash," Silive.com, accessed July 4, 2017, http://www.silive.com/news/2010/07/staten_island_ferry_excaptain.html

[23] Meier, Barry. "Pain Pills Add Cost and Delays to Job Injuries," The New York Times, accessed July 4, 2017, http://www.nytimes.com/2012/06/03/health/painkillers-add-costs-and-delays-to-workplace-injuries.html

[24] Bachhuber, Marcus A., MD, MSHP et al. "Increasing Benzodiazepine Prescriptions and Overdose Mortality in the United States, 1996–2013," American Journal of Public Health, April 2016, accessed January 17, 2018, doi: 10.2105/ AJPH.2016.303061

[25] Grohol, John. "Top 25 Psychiatric Medications for 2016," PsychCentral, accessed February 14, 2018, https://psychcentral.com/blog/top-25-psychiatric-medications-for-2016/

[26] Ornstein, Charles and Ryann Grochowski Jones, "One Nation, Under Sedation: Medicare Paid for Nearly 40 Million Tranquilizer Prescriptions in 2013," ProPublica, accessed January 4, 2018, https://www.propublica.org/article/medicare-paid-for-nearly-40-million-tranquilizer-prescriptions-in-2013

[27] Chase, Dave. "City Slashes Healthcare Costs by Improving Health Benefits," Forbes, February 8, 2016, accessed July 4, 2017, https://www.forbes.com/sites/davechase/2016/02/08/city-slashes-healthcare-costs-by-improving-health-benefits

[28] Fenton, Joshua J., MD, MPH et al. "The Cost of Satisfaction: A National Study of Patient Satisfaction, Health Care Utilization, Expenditures, and Mortality."

[29] Roy, Avik. "If Republicans Delay the Cadillac Tax, They Will Cost Taxpayers Far More in the Long Run," Forbes, accessed March 26, 2018, https://www.forbes.com/sites/theapothecary/2015/12/11/if-republicans-delay-the-cadillac-tax-they-will-cost-taxpayers-far-more-in-the-long-run

[30] "Health Care Costs: A Primer," The Henry J. Kaiser Family Foundation, accessed July 4, 2016, http://www.kff.org/report-section/health-care-costs-a-primer-2012-report/

[31] Sussman, Anna Louie. "Burden of Health-Care Costs Moves to the Middle Class," The Wall Street Journal, accessed December 12, 2016, https://www.wsj.com/articles/burden-of-health-care-costs-moves-to-the-middle-class-1472166246

[32] Auerbach, David I. and Arthur L. Kellermann. "How Does Growth in Health Care Costs Affect the American Family?" accessed July 4, 2016, https://www.rand.org/pubs/research_briefs/RB9605.html

[33] Idowu, Modupe. "Premium Hikes Eat Up Teacher Pay Raise," accessed October 14, 2016, http://mynbc15.com/news/local/premium-hikes-eat-up-teacher-pay-raise

[34] "Make America Make Again: Manufacturing in the U.S.A.," WAMU/NPR., accessed February 1, 2017, http://the1a.org/shows/2017-01-25/made-in-america

[35] Ritholtz, Barry. "Health-Care Costs Ate Your Pay Raises," Bloomberg, accessed November 5, 2016, https://www.bloomberg.com/view/articles/2016-09-28/health-care-costs-ate-your-pay-raises

[36] Welch, Ashley. "Drug Overdoses Killed More Americans Last Year Than the Vietnam War," CBS News, accessed March 26, 2018, https://www.cbsnews.com/news/opioids-drug-overdose-killed-more-americans-last-year-than-the-vietnam-war/

[37] Labott, Kristin. An Unlikely Addict. CreateSpace, 2015

[38] Young, Richard A. and Jennifer E. DeVoe, "Who Will Have Health Insurance in the Future? An Updated Projection," Annals Family Medicine 10(2010): 2 accessed July 4, 2016, doi:10.1370/afm.1348

[39] Huddleston, Cameron. "69% of Americans Have Less Than $1,000 in Savings," accessed November 4, 2016, https://www.gobankingrates.com/personal-finance/data-americans-savings/

[40] Lamontagne, Christina. "NerdWallet Health finds Medical Bankruptcy accounts for majority of personal bankruptcies," accessed July 4, 2016, https://www.nerdwallet.com/blog/health/medical-bankruptcy/

[41] Woolley, Suzanne. "American Health Care Tragedies Are Taking Over Crowdfunding," Bloomberg, accessed July 4, 2017 https://www.bloomberg.com/news/articles/2017-06-12/americas-health-care-crisis-is-a-gold-mine-for-crowdfunding

[42] "List of Figures in 2013 Cost Trends Report by the Health Policy Commission," Health Policy Commission, accessed July 4, 2016, http://www.mass.gov/anf/docs/hpc/2013-ctr-chartbook.pdf

[43] Brink, Susan. "How Health Care Costs Affect Small Town Living," U.S. News, accessed July 4, 2016, https://health.usnews.com/health-news/hos-pital-of-tomorrow/articles/2014/02/05/how-health-care-costs-affect-small-town-living

[44] James, John. "A New, Evidence-based Estimate of Patient Harms Associated with Hospital Care" Journal of Patient Safety 9(2013): 3, accessed July 4, 2016, doi:10.1097/PTS.0b013e3182948a69; "Medical Errors Are No. 3 Cause of U.S Deaths, Researchers Say," NPR: Boise State Public Radio, accessed July 4, 2016, http://www.npr.org/sections/health-shots/2016/05/03/476636183/death-certificates-undercount-toll-of-medical-errors; "Study Suggests Medical Errors Now Third Leading Cause of Death in the U.S.," John Hopkins Medicine, accessed July 4, 2017, https://www.hopkinsmedicine.org/news/media/releases/study_suggests_medical_errors_now_third_leading_cause_of_death_in_the_us

[45] Eunjung Cha, Ariana. "Researchers: Medical Errors Now Third Leading Cause of Death in United States," The Washington Post, May 3, 2016, accessed July 4, 2016, https://www.washingtonpost.com/news/to-your-health/wp/2016/05/03/researchers-medical-errors-now-third-leading-cause-of-death-in-united-states/

[46] Krakauer, Jon. Where Men Win Glory: The Odyssey of Pat Tillman. (New York: Doubleday, 2010), 343; "United States Military Casualties of War," Wikipedia, accessed July 4, 2017, https://en.wikipedia.org/wiki/United_States_mili- tary_casualties_of_war

[47] Kliff, Sarah. "Do No Harm," Vox, accessed July 4, 2016, http://www.vox.com/2015/7/9/8905959/medical-harm-infection-prevention

[48] Makary, Marty. Unaccountable: What Hospitals Won't Tell You and How Transparency Can Revolutionize Health Care, London: Bloomsbury, 2012

[49] For this calculation, I compared actual health care premium growth rates with historical rates of inflation, then assumed the difference would have been invested in an S&P index fund and that dividends would have been reinvested.

[50] "Retirement Plan Access and Participation Across Generations," The Pew Charitable Trusts, accessed March 2, 2017, http://www.pewtrusts. org/en/research-and-analysis/issue-briefs/2017/02/retirement-plan-access-and-participation-across-generations; Williams, Sean. "Nearly 7 in 10 Americans Have Less Than $1,000 in Savings," USA Today, accessed March 2, 2017, https://www.usatoday.com/story/money/personalfinance/2016/10/09/savings-study/91083712/

[51] Cabbabe, Samer. "The Medical Profession Has a Bad Reputation. Here's Why," Kevin MD, accessed March 1, 2017, http://www.kevinmd.com/blog/2017/03/medical-profession-bad-reputation-heres.html

[52] Sinsky, Christine, MD et al. "Allocation of Physician Time in Ambulatory Practice: A Time and Motion Study in 4 Specialties," Annals of Internal Medicine 165(2016): 11, accessed January 4, 2016, DOI: 10.7326/M16-0961

[53] Boodman, Sandra. "Patients Lose When Doctors Can't Do Good Physical Exams," Kaiser Health News, accessed July 4, 2016, http://khn.org/news/patients-lose-when-doctors-do-not-perform-physical-exams-correctly/

[54] Christine Sinsky, M.D. et al., "Allocation of Physician Time in Ambulatory Practice: A Time and Motion Study in 4 Specialties."

[55] Murray, Ken. "How Doctors Die" Saturday Evening Post, April 2013, accessed July 4, 2016, http://www.saturdayeveningpost.com/2013/03/06/in-the-magazine/health-in-the-magazine/how-doctors-die.html

[56] Hatkoff, Craig, Rabbi Irwin Kula, and Zach Levine. "How to Die in America: Welcome to La Crosse, Wisconsin" Forbes, accessed July 4, 2016, https://www.forbes.com/sites/offwhitepapers/2014/09/23/how-to-die-in-america-welcome-to-la-crosse/#17df59bbe8c6

[57] Epstein, David & Propublica, "When Evidence Says No, but Doctors Say Yes," The Atlantic, accessed March 2, 2018, https://www.theatlantic.com/health/archive/2017/02/when-evidence-says-no-but-doctors-say-yes/517368/

[58] Kolata, Gina. "Why 'Useless' Surgery Is Still Popular," The New York Times, accessed July 4, 2016, https://www.nytimes.com/2016/08/04/upshot/the-right-to-know-that-an-operation-is-next-to-useless.html

[59] "Infographic: Health Care Waste," PBS News Hour, accessed July 4, 2016, https://www.pbs.org/newshour/spc/multimedia/health-750b/

[60] This chart is adapted from one provided to me by an industry insider.

[61] "How Many Doctors Does It Take to Start a Healthcare Revolution? Full Transcript," Freakonomics, accessed July 9, 2016, http://freakonomics.com/2015/04/09/-how-many-doctors-does-it-take-to-start-a-healthcare-revolution-full-transcript/

[62] Gawande, Atul. "The Hot Spotters," The New Yorker, accessed July 4, 2016, http://www.newyorker.com/magazine/2011/01/24/the-hot-spotters

[63] This data comes from ClearHealthCosts internal datasets that they've given us permission to use.

[64] "Employer Health Benefits," The Kaiser Family Foundation and Health Research & Educational Trust, accessed July 4, 2016, https://kaiserfamily-foundation.files.wordpress.com/2013/04/7936.pdf

[65] This data comes from ClearHealthCosts internal datasets that they've given us permission to use.

[66] Private discussions with other industry executives and experts not for attribution.

[67] "Fraud, Waste and Abuse in Social Services: Identifying and Overcoming This Modern-Day Epidemic," Accenture Consulting, accessed March 2, 2017, https://www.accenture.com/us-en/insight-fraud-waste-abuse-social-services-summary

[68] Private discussions with other industry executives and experts not for attribution.

[69] "HRI Benefits Advisor Compensation Disclosure Form," Health Rosetta, accessed May 25, 2017, https://healthrosetta.org/learn/benefits-advisor-disclosure/

[70] Fry, Richard. "Millennials Surpass Gen Xers as the Largest Generation in U.S. Labor Force," Pew Research Center, accessed January 18, 2018, http://www.pewre-search.org/fact-tank/2015/05/11/millennials-surpass-gen-xers-as-the-largest-generation-in-us-labor-force/

[71] Goldhill, David. Catastrophic Care: Why Everything We Think We Know about Heath Care Is Wrong New York: Knopf Doubleday Publishing Group, 2013

[72] Hidalgo, Jason. "Here's How Millennials Could Change Health Care" USA Today, accessed February 7, 2018, http://www.usatoday.com/story/news/politics/elections/2016/02/07/heres-how-millennials-could-change-health-care/79818756/

[73] "The Future Health Ecosystem Today," Cascadia Capital, accessed January 15, 2016, http://www.cascadiacapital.com/story/cascadias-digital-healt-care-team-releases-the-future-of-healthcare-today-report/

[74] Crichton, Danny. "Millennials Are Destroying Banks, and It's the Banks' Fault," TechCrunch, accessed February 15, 2018, https://techcrunch.com/2015/05/30/millennial-banks/

[75] Hanft, Adam. "The Stunning Evolution of Millennials: They've Become the Ben Franklin Generation," THE BLOG Huffington Post, accessed January 11, 2017, http://www.huffingtonpost.com/adam-hanft/the-stunning-evolution-of_b_6108412.html

[76] Crichton, Danny. "Millennials Are Destroying Banks, and It's the Banks' Fault."

[77] Farr, Christina. "Are Millennials Ready to Ditch Their Regular Doctor?" KQED Science, accessed July 4, 2017), http://ww2.kqed.org/futureofyou/2015/08/12/convenience-or-loyalty-what-do-millennials-value-more-when-it-comes-to-their-health

[78] "Growing Retail Clinic Industry Employs, Empowers Nurse Practitioners," Robert Wood Johnson Foundation, accessed July 4, 2016, http://www.rwjf.org/en/library/articles-and-news/2015/02/growing-retail-clinic-industry-employs--empowers-nurse-practitio.html; Pollack, Craig E., et al. "The Growth of Retail Clinics and the Medical Home: Two Trends in Concert or in Conflict?" Health Affairs (29): 5, accessed July 4 2016, doi: 10.1377/hlthaff.2010.0089; Jaspen, Bruce. "Retail Clinics Hit 10 Million Annual Visits but Just 2% of Primary Care Market," Forbes, accessed July 4, 2016, https://www.forbes.com/sites/brucejapsen/2015/04/23/retail-clinics-hit-10-million-annual-visits-but-just-2-of-primary-care-market

[79] Hidalgo, Jason. "Here's How Millennials Could Change Health Care"

[80] "People Love Their Health Benefits. But Do They Understand Them?" Collective Health (2016), https://collectivehealth.com/insights/consumer-health-benefits-survey-2015/

[81] Hidalgo, Jason. "Here's How Millennials Could Change Health Care"

[82] Dews, Fred. "Brookings Data Now: 75 Percent of 2025 Workforce Will Be Millennials," accessed July 4, 2016, https://www.brookings.edu/blog/brookings-now/2014/07/17/brookings-data-now-75-percent-of-2025-workforce-will-be-millennials/; Mitchell, Alastair. "The Rise of the Millennial Workforce," Wired, accessed May 25, 2017, https://www.wired.com/insights/2013/08/the-rise-of-the-millennial-workforce/

[83] "Freelancers Now Make Up 35% Of U.S. Workforce," Forbes, accessed June 25, 2018, https://www.forbes.com/sites/elainepofeldt/2016/10/06/new-survey-freelance-economy-shows-rapid-growth

[84] "A Conversation with Surgeon, Author, and Researcher Atul Gawande," Filmed June 2018 The Aspen Institute - Aspen Ideas Festival, Aspen CO, https://www.youtube.com/watch?v=_kaB8UL_TNk&feature=youtu.be

[85] "Obamacare plans get more restrictive and deductibles get pricier in 2018," CNBC, accessed June 25, 2018, https://www.cnbc.com/2017/11/30/obamacare-plans-get-narrower-and-deductibles-get-pricier-in-2018.html

[86] "The Price of Excess, Identifying Waste in Health Care Spending," Price waterhouse Coopers' Health Research Institute, accessed January 22, 2017, http://www.oss.net/dynamaster/file_archive/080509/59f26a38c114f2295757bb-6be522128a/The%20Price%20of%20Excess%20-%20Identifying%20Waste%20in%20Healthcare%20Spending%20-%20PWC.pdf

[87] Cothran, Josh. "US Health Care Spending: Who Pays?" California Health Care Foundation, accessed November 5, 2017, http://www.chcf.org/publi-cations/2014/07/data-viz-hcc-national

[88] Kocher, Robert, MD and Nikhil R. Sahni, BS. "Rethinking Health Care Labor" The New England Journal of Medicine (2011): 365, accessed July 4, 2016, doi: 10.1056/NEJMp1109649

[89] Ibid.

[90] Dayen, David. "The Hidden Monopolies That Raise Drug Prices," The American Prospect Longform, accessed May 17, 2017, http://prospect.org/article/hidden-monopolies-raise-drug-prices; Hemphill, Thomas. "The "Troubles" with Pharmacy Benefit Managers," CATO Institute, accessed June 1, 2017, https://object.cato.org/sites/cato.org/files/serials/files/regulation/2017/3/regulation-v40n1-5.pdf

[91] Thomas, Tim. "Your PBM Adds Drugs Like Duexis to Your Formulary; Why Should You Have to Pay?" Crystal Clear Rx, accessed March 2, 2017, http://crystalclearrx.com/your-pbm-adds-drugs-duexis-your-formulary-why-should-you-have-pay

[92] Flores, Mark. "United Health Care Administered ERISA Plan Sued for Embezzlement in Medical Claims Overpayment Offset Dispute," AVYM, accessed July 4, 2016, http://avym.com/united-healthcare-administered-er-isa-plan-sued-for-embezzlement-in-medical-claims-overpayment-offset-dis-pute/

[93] Parker-Pope, Tara. "How Doctors and Patients Do Harm" New York Times Well, accessed December 12, 2017, https://well.blogs.nytimes.com/2012/04/20/how-doctors-and-patients-do-harm/

[94] Ducharme, Jamie. "Misdiagnosing Cancer Is More Common Than We Think" Boston Wellness, accessed January 22, 2018, http://www.bostonmagazine.com/health/blog/2013/01/31/study-cancer-misdiagnose/

[95] Greene, Dr. Alan. "Jumping Out of a Plane More Than 47 Times Safer Than Checking into a Hospital. Unless…" Dr. Greene's Blog, January 27, 2018, https://www.drgreene.com/jumping-plane-47-times-safer-checking-hospital/

[96] "Top Industries," OpenSecrets.org, accessed, July 4, 2017, https://www.opensecrets.org/lobby/top.php?indexType=i

[97] "Leapfrog Hospital Safety Grade," http://www.hospitalsafetygrade.org/

[98] "Hospital Compare," Medicare.gov, accessed July 4 2016, https://www.medicare.gov/hospitalcompare

[99] "HR Consulting in the US: Market Research Report," IBISWorld, accessed June 3, 2017, https://www.ibisworld.com/industry-trends/market-research-reports/professional-scientific-technical-services/professional-scientific-technical-services/hr-consulting.html

[100] Dendy, Michael. "The OPEC of Healthcare," LinkedIn, accessed July 4, 2016, https://www.linkedin.com/pulse/opec-healthcare-michael-mike-dendy

[101] Dunlap, Rod. "Robotic Process Automation: A Better Way to Boost Auto-Adjudication Rates," hfma, accessed July 4, 2016, https://www.hfma.org/Content.aspx?id=48424, The number cited here is 80%, but multiple industry insiders have told me it's more like 90+% in private conversations.

[102] Private discussions with other industry executives and experts not for attribution.

[103] "Fraud, Waste and Abuse in Social Services: Identifying and Overcoming This Modern-Day Epidemic," Accenture Consulting.

[104] Rayman, Noah. "The World's Top 5 Cybercrime Hotspots," Time, accessed July 4, 2016, http://time.com/3087768/the-worlds-5-cyber-crime-hotspots/

[105] Rashid, Fahmida. "Why Hackers Want Your Health Care Data Most of

All," InfoWorld, accessed July 4, 2016, http://www.infoworld.com/article/2983634/security/why-hackers-want-your-health-care-data-breaches-most-of-all.html

[106] The Nilson Report (October 2016): 1096, accessed January 17, 2017, https://www.nilsonreport.com/upload/content_promo/The_Nilson_Report_10-17-2016.pdf; Kiernan, John. "Credit Card & Debit Card Fraud Statistics," WalletHub, accessed March 2, 2017, https://wallethub.com/edu/credit-debit-card-fraud-statistics/25725/

[107] Private discussions with other industry executives and experts not for attribution.

[108] Pollitz, Karen and Matthew Rae. "Workplace Wellness Programs Characteristics and Requirements," The Henry J. Kaiser Family Foundation, accessed July 4, 2016, https://www.kff.org/private-insurance/issue-brief/workplace-wellness-programs-characteristics-and-requirements/; Fry, Erika. "Corporate Wellness Programs: Healthy or Hokey?" Fortune Health, accessed February 10, 2018, http://fortune.com/2017/03/15/corporate-health-wellness-programs/

[109] Kuraitis, Vince. "A Founding Father of DM Astonishingly Declares: 'My Kid is Ugly,'" e-CareManagement Blog, http://e-caremanagement.com/a-founding-father-of-dm-astonishingly-declares-my-kid-is-ugly/

[110] O'Donnell, Michael. "My Last Lecture," American Journal of Health Promotion (2016): 30, accessed January 3, 2017, doi: 10.1177/0890117116671802

[111] Anderson, L.V. "Workplace Wellness Programs Are a Sham," Slate, accessed November 5, 2016, http://www.slate.com/articles/health_and_science/the_ladder/2016/09/workplace_wellness_programs_are_a_sham.html, Note the 13,000 shares on Facebook alone.

[112] "About the USPSTF," U.S. Preventive Services, accessed March 2, 2017, https://www.uspreventiveservicestaskforce.org/Page/Name/about-the-uspstf

[113] "Health Checkups: When You Need Them—And When You Don't," Choosing Wisely, accessed July 4, 2016, http://www.choosingwisely.org/patient-resources/health-checkups/

[114] Lewis, Al. "The 401W: A Wellness Program Even Al Lewis Could Love," The Health Care Blog, accessed July 4, 2017, http://thehealthcareblog.com/blog/2017/04/17/the-401w-a-wellness-program-even-al-lewis-could-love/

[115] Lewis, Al. "A Wellness Program Everyone Can Love," Insurance Thought Leadership, accessed May 17, 2017, http://insurancethoughtleadership.com/a-wellness-program-everyone-can-love/

[116] Fry, Erika. "Corporate Wellness Programs: Healthy or Hokey?"

[117] Burjek, Andie. "Health Literacy Empowers Employees to Make Better Decisions," Workforce, accessed July 4, 2017, http://www.workforce.com/2017/02/07/health-literacy-empowers-employees-make-better-decisions/

[118] "IOM Report: Estimated $750B Wasted Annually in Health Care System," Kaiser Health News, Accessed July 4, 2016, http://khn.org/morning-breakout/iom-report/; "The Price of Excess, Identifying Waste in Healthcare Spending." PricewaterhouseCoopers Health Research Institute

[119] Wallace, Jean E. et al. "Physician Wellness: A Missing Quality Indicator," The Lancet 374: 9702, accessed July 4, 2016, doi: https://doi.org/10.1016/S0140-6736(09)61424-0

[120] Kenney, Charles. "Better, Faster, More Affordable," Seattle Business, accessed July 4, 2016, http://seattlebusinessmag.com//article/better-faster-more-affordable

[121] Kolata, Gina. "Why 'Useless' Surgery Is Still Popular."

[122] The 67 percent number cited here is from a transparent broker based on his own experience. It's consistent with what I've encountered from many others.

[123] "Employer Health Benefits," The Kaiser Family Foundation and Health Research & Educational Trust; This represents the average premium inflation rate from 2000-2009 based on the figures provided in the Kaiser/HRET 2009 Employer Health Benefits Annual Survey.

[124] "Influence & Lobbying / Lobbying / Top Industries," Open Secrets.org, accessed February 28, 2018, https://www.opensecrets.org/lobby/top.php?indexType=i

[125] Parkinson, Jay. "Toward a New Definition of Primary Care: Primary Care 3.0." Jay Parkinson MD Blog, accessed July 4, 2017, https://blog.jayparkinsonmd.com/2017/06/20/toward-a-new-definition-of-primary-care-primary-care-3-0/

[126] "Influence & Lobbying / Lobbying / Top Industries," Open Secrets.org, accessed February 28, 2018, https://www.opensecrets.org/lobby/top.php?indexType=i

[127] "India's Philanthropist-Surgeon Delivers Cardiac Care Henry Ford-Style,"

NPR: Boise State Public Radio, accessed July 4, 2016, http://www.npr.org/sections/goatsandsoda/2015/01/05/375142025/indias-philanthropist-de-livers-cardiac-surgery-henry-ford-style

[128] Thomas, Katie. "His Doctors Were Stumped. Then He Took Over," The New York Times, accessed July 4, 2017, http://mobile.nytimes.com/2017/02/04/business/his-doctors-were-stumped-then-he-took-over.html

[129] Main, Tom and Adrian Slywotzky. "Volume-to-Value Revolution," accessed July 4, 2016, http://www.oliverwyman.com/our-expertise/insights/2012/nov/the-volume-to-value-revolution.html

[130] Chase, Dave. "Privia Leads $1.2 Billion Primary Care Renaissance Enabling Economic Renewal," accessed July 4, 2016, http://www.forbes.com/sites/davechase/2016/05/05/privia-leads-1-2-billion-primary-care-renais-sance-enabling-economic-renewal

[131] Chase, Dave. "Hospital CEOs Behaving Badly and the Devastating Consequences on the Middle Class," accessed July 4, 2017, http://www.forbes.com/sites/davechase/2016/08/29/hospital-ceos-behaving-badly-the-dev-astating-consequences-on-the-middle-class/

[132] Chase, Dave. "Healthcare CEOs Making Newspaper Industry Mistakes," Forbes, accessed July4,2016, http://www.forbes.com/sites/davechase/2012/02/09/healthcare-ceos-guide-to-avoiding-newspaper-in-dustry-mistakes

[133] Damania, Zubin. "Lose Yourself," ZDogg MD, accessed July 4, 2016, http://zdoggmd.com/lose-yourself/

[134] Chase, Dave. "City Slashes Healthcare Costs by Improving Health Benefits," Forbes, accessed July 4, 2016, http://www.forbes.com/sites/davechase/2016/02/08/city-slashes-healthcare-costs-by-improving-health-benefits

[135] Damania, Zubin. "Lose Yourself," ZDogg MD, accessed July 4, 2016, http://zdoggmd.com/lose-yourself/

[136] Chase, Dave. "Economic Development 3.0: Playing the Health Card," accessed January 30, 2017, https://www.linkedin.com/pulse/economic-de-velopment-30-playing-health-card-dave-chase

[137] Parkinson, Jay. "Toward a New Definition of Primary Care: Primary Care 3.0." Jay Parkinson MD Blog, accessed July 4, 2017, https://blog.jayparkins-onmd.com/2017/06/20/toward-a-new-definition-of-primary-care-primary-

care-3-0/

[138] Julapalli, Venu. "The Tenets of Health 3.0," Tinture.io, accessed July 4, 2017, http://tincture.io/the-tenets-of-health-3-0-516e51e3e89f#.k71j0vv45

[139] "India's Philanthropist-Surgeon Delivers Cardiac Care Henry Ford-Style," NPR: Boise State Public Radio, accessed July 4, 2016, http://www.npr.org/sections/goatsandsoda/2015/01/05/375142025/indias-philanthropist-delivers-cardiac-surgery-henry-ford-style

[140] Thomas, Katie. "His Doctors Were Stumped. Then He Took Over," The New York Times, accessed July 4, 2017, http://mobile.nytimes.com/2017/02/04/business/his-doctors-were-stumped-then-he-took-over.html

[141] Main, Tom and Adrian Slywotzky. "Volume-to-Value Revolution," accessed July 4, 2016, http://www.oliverwyman.com/our-expertise/insights/2012/nov/the-volume-to-value-revolution.html

[142] Chase, Dave. "Privia Leads $1.2 Billion Primary Care Renaissance Enabling Economic Renewal," accessed July 4, 2016, http://www.forbes.com/sites/davechase/2016/05/05/privia-leads-1-2-billion-primary-care-renaissance-enabling-economic-renewal

[143] Chase, Dave. "Hospital CEOs Behaving Badly and the Devastating Consequences on the Middle Class," accessed July 4, 2017, http://www.forbes.com/sites/davechase/2016/08/29/hospital-ceos-behaving-badly-the-devastating-consequences-on-the-middle-class/

[144] Chase, Dave. "Healthcare CEOs Making Newspaper Industry Mistakes," accessed July 4, 2016, http://www.forbes.com/sites/davechase/2012/02/09/healthcare-ceos-guide-to-avoiding-newspaper-industry-mistakes

[145] Damania, Zubin. "Lose Yourself," ZDogg MD, accessed July 4, 2016, http://zdoggmd.com/lose-yourself/

[146] 146 Chase, Dave. "City Slashes Healthcare Costs by Improving Health Benefits," Forbes, accessed July 4, 2016, http://www.forbes.com/sites/davechase/2016/02/08/city-slashes-healthcare-costs-by-improving-health-benefits

[147] Booske, Bridget C. et al. "County Health Rankings Working Paper: Different Perspectives for Assigning Weights to Determinants of Health," accessed July 4, 2016, http://www.countyhealthrankings.org/sites/default/files/differentPerspectivesForAssigningWeightsToDeterminantsOfHealth.pdf

[148] Chase, Dave. "Economic Development 3.0: Playing the Health Card," accessed January 30, 2017, https://www.linkedin.com/pulse/economic-de-

velopment-30-playing-health-card-dave-chase

[149] Sussman, Anna Louie. "Burden of Health-Care Costs Moves to the Middle Class."

[150] "athenahealth Partners with Affected Florida Community to Combat Zika Virus," athenahealth, accessed July 4, 2017, http://newsroom.athenahealth. com/phoenix.zhtml?c=253091&p=irol-newsArticle&ID=2192379

[151] Kocher, Bob. "How I Was Wrong About ObamaCare"; Diamond, Dan. "Pulse Check: Confessions of an Ex-Regulator on How Government Should Work," Politico, accessed July 4, 2016, http://www.politico.com/story/2016/05/ confessions-of-an-ex-regulator-farzad-mostashari-on-how-government-should-work-222901

[152] Based on a personal interview with Dr. Paul Grundy, IBM's Chief Medical Officer & Global Director of Healthcare Transformation

[153] Gould, Elise. "2014 Continues a 35-Year Trend of Broad-Based Wage Stagnation." EPI analysis of Current Population Survey Outgoing Rotation Group microdata, Economic Policy Institute, accessed April 27, 2018, https://www. epi.org/publication/stagnant-wages-in-2014/

[154] Graphic courtesy of Dr. Paul Grundy, IBM's Chief Medical Officer and Director of Health Care Transformation IBM Health Care Life Science Industry.

[155] Cothran, Josh. "US Health Care Spending: Who Pays?"

[156] "How Many Doctors Does It Take to Start a Healthcare Revolution? Full Transcript," Freakonomics, accessed July 4, 2017, http://freakonomics. com/2015/04/09/how-many-doctors-does-it-take-to-start-a-healthcare-revolution-full-transcript/

[157] Keckley, Paul, PhD. "Keynote: Health Reform 2.0: What's Ahead?," filmed March 2015, 4:02, https://www.youtube.com/watch?v=m4cZ4kZw8-E&feature=youtu.be&t=4m2s

[158] "When a Hospital Closes: What Really Happens to the Patients Left Behind?" Advisory Board, accessed November 5, 2017, http://www.advisory.com/daily-briefing/2015/05/06/when-a-hospital-closes-what-really-happens-to-the-patients-left-behind

[159] "Study: 7 of 10 Most Profitable US Hospitals Are Nonprofits," AP News, accessed November5, 2017, https://apnews.com/8867beb-032c049378e4a83d-150cb8bc3

[160] Herman, Bob. "Hospitals Are Making a Fortune on Wall Street," Axios, accessed December 10, 2017, https://www.axios.com/hospitals-are-making-a-fortune-on-wall-street-2513530266.html

[161] Galewitz, Phil and Anna Gorman, "More Ailing Hospitals Are Being Resuscitated as Upscale Living Spaces," The Washington Post, accessed December 7, 2017, https://www.washingtonpost.com/realestate/more-ailing-hospitals-are-being-resuscitated-as-upscale-living-spaces/2017/11/21/e1af7ec2-b34f-11e7-9e58-e6288544af98_story.html

[162] Kaysen, Ronda. "Repurposing Closed Hospitals as For-Profit Medical Malls," The New York Times, accessed November 5, 2017, https://www.nytimes.com/2014/03/05/realestate/commercial/repurposing-closed-hospitals-as-for-profit-medical-malls.html

[163] Woodard, Colin. "The Coolest Shipyard in America," Politico Magazine, accessed February 17, 2018, https://www.politico.com/magazine/story/2016/07/philadelphia-what-works-navy-yard-214072

[164] Chase, Dave. "VP HR & Benefits Should Get Big Bonuses for Saving 50-90% on Big Ticket Healthcare," LinkedIn, accessed September 28, 2014, https://www.linkedin.com/pulse/20140928130122-255656-vp-hr-benefits-should-get-big-bonuses-saving-50-90-on-big-ticket-healthcare/

[165] St. John, Allen. "How the Affordable Care Act Drove Down Personal Bankruptcy - Expanded Health Insurance Helped Cut the Number of Filings by Half," Consumer Reports, accessed February 28, 2018 https://www.consumerreports.org/personal-bankruptcy/how-the-acadrove-down-personal-bankruptcy/

[166] Mitchell, Jerry and The (Jackson, Miss.) Clarion Ledger. "Opioid Makers Face Hundreds of Lawsuits for Misleading Doctors about Drug's Addictive Nature," USA Today, accessed March 26, 2018, https://www.usatoday.com/story/news/nation-now/2018/01/29/judge-stop-legal-fights-and-curb-opioid-epidemic/1072798001/

[167] "The Underestimated Cost of the Opioid Crisis." The Council of Economic Advisers, accessed March 20, 2018, https://www.whitehouse.gov/sites/whitehouse.gov/files/images/The%20Underestimated%20Cost%20of%20the%20Opioid%20Crisis.pdf

[168] "The $272 Billion Swindle: Why Thieves Love America's Health-Care System." The Economist, accessed March 26, 2018, https://www.economist.com/news/united-states/21603078-why-thieves-love-americas-health-care-system-272-billion-swindle

[169] "A Substance Use Cost Calculator for Employers." National Safety Council, accessed March 20, 2018, https://forms.nsc.org/substance-use-employer-calculator/index.aspx

[170] Goplerud, Eric, Sarah Hodge, and Tess Benham. "A Substance Use Cost Calculator for US Employers with an Emphasis on Prescription Pain Medication Misuse," Journal of Occupational and Environmental Medicine, 2017 Nov, 59(11): 1063–1071.https://dx.doi.org/10.1097%2FJOM.0000000000001157

[171] "Medication Assisted Treatment & Direct Primary Care," Bluegrass Family Wellness, accessed March 20, 2018, http://www.bluegrassfamilywellness.com/home-recovery/

[172] "Vera Whole Health Achieves Validation Endorsement by Care Innovations™ Validation Institute" accessed April 27, 2018, https://www.prnewswire.com/news-releases/vera-whole-health-achieves-validation-endorsement-by-care-innovations-validation-institute-300598404.html

[173] "Pennsylvania Rural Health Model," Centers for Medicare & Medicaid Services, accessed March 20, 2018, https://innovation.cms.gov/initiatives/pa-rural-health-model/

[174] Armstrong, David. "Secret Trove Reveals Bold 'Crusade' to Make Oxycontin a Blockbuster," STAT News, accessed March 27, 2018, https://www.statnews.com/2016/09/22/abbott-oxycontin-crusade/

[175] Wagner, Tony. "ADrugmaker Used 'The Wizard of Oz' to Sell OxyContin," Marketplace, accessed March 27, 2018 https://www.marketplace.org/2017/12/15/health-care/uncertain-hour/drugmaker-used-wizard-oz-sell-oxycontin

[176] "The $272 billion swindle," The Economist, accessed July 4, 2017, https://www.economist.com/united-states/2014/05/31/the-272-billion-swindle

[177] "IOM Report: Estimated $750B Wasted Annually in Health Care System," Kaiser Health News.

[178] "DOL Files Suit Against Macy's for Alleged Health and Welfare Plan Violations," haynesboone, accessed October 1, 2017, https://blogs.haynesboone.com/2017/09/20/dol-files-suit-macys-alleged-health-welfare-plan-violations/

[179] "The $272 billion swindle," The Economist.

[180] Jen Wieczner, "Most Millennials Think They'll Be Worse Off Than Their Parents," Fortune, accessed August 14, 2017, http://fortune.com/2016/03/01/millennials-worse-parents-retirement/ refers to this study

[181] David Goldhill, Catastrophic Care: Why Everything We Think We Know about Health Care Is Wrong (New York: Knopf Doubleday Publishing Group, 2013)

[182] Dan Munro, U.S. Healthcare Actually Isn't Broken, Insurance Thought Leadership, accessed August 15, 2017, http://insurancethoughtleadership.com/u-s-healthcare-actually-isnt-broken/

[183] "Joanne Disch testifying on Patient Safety" C-SPAN, accessed August 15, 2017, https://www.c-span.org/video/?c4507180/joanne-disch-testifying-patient-safety deaths; John T. James, PhD, "A New, Evidence-based Estimate of Patient Harms Associated with Hospital Care" Journal of Patient Safety (September 2013): 122-28, accessed August, 15 2017, http://journals.lww.com/journalpatientsafety/Fulltext/2013/09000/A_New,_Evidence_based_Estimate_of_Patient_Harms.2.aspx

[184] Dan Kopf, "The opioid crisis is driving up deaths of millennials in the US," Quartz, accessed June 18, 2018, https://qz.com/1169672/us-millennials-were-almost-20-more-likely-to-die-in-2016-than-2014/

[185] "The Art of Personomics," John Hopkins Medicine, accessed July 4, 2017, http://www.hopkinscim.org/breakthrough/summer-2015/the-art-of-personomics/

[186] "Health Insurance's Bunker Buster," Huffington Post, accessed June 25, 2018 https://www.huffingtonpost.com/dave-chase/health-insurances-bunker_b_600587.html

[187] "10 Mistakes Amazon, Berkshire Hathaway and J.P. Morgan Must Avoid to Make a Dent in Healthcare," LinkedIn Pulse, accessed June 25, 2018, https://www.linkedin.com/pulse/10-mistakes-amazon-berkshire-hathaway-jp-morgan-must-avoid-dave-chase/

[188] "NSC Poll: 99% of Doctors Prescribe Opioids Longer than CDC Recommends," WorkCompWire, accessed June 25, 2018, https://www.workcompwire.com/2016/03/nsc-poll-99-of-doctors-prescribe-opioids-longer-than-cdc-recommends/

[189] "Healthcare 'Tax' Has Crushed Nest Eggs By $1,000,000 Per Household," Forbes, accessed June 25, 2018, https://www.forbes.com/sites/davechase/2015/05/27/health-care-tax-has-crushed-nest-eggs-by-1000000-per-household

[190] "Health Plan Industry's Worst Nightmare: Employers Realizing They Are Actually The Insurance Company," Forbes, accessed June 25, 2018,

https://www.forbes.com/sites/davechase/2016/04/19/health-plan-industrys-worst-nightmare-employers-realizing-they-are-actually-the-insurance-company/#6b49260e7556

[191] "End Predatory Healthcare Pricing," Change.org, accessed June 25, 2018, https://www.change.org/p/end-predatory-healthcare-pricing

[192] "New Study: Many Hospital Closings May Have Little Effect on Local Health," Nonprofit Quarterly, accessed June 25, 2018, https://nonprofitquarterly.org/2015/05/11/new-study-many-hospital-closings-may-have-little-effect-on-local-health/

[193] Laura Santhanam, "1 million Americans pool money in religious ministries to pay for health care," accessed July 4, 2018, https://www.pbs.org/newshour/health/1-million-americans-pool-money-in-religious-ministries-to-pay-for-health-care

.

INDEX

and evidence-based
management programs,
135–136
example of, 66–67
and primary care physicians, 201
as revenue generator, 77–78
and wellness programs, 102–104
OxyContin, 4

P

pain clinics, 8
pain management, 3, 6–7, 12,
215–216
Parkinson, Jay, 179
patient volume, 5
patient-centered medical home
(PCMH), 200
pay and chase insurance programs,
55, 96–97, 99
payment integrity technology, 99,
199
PBM (Pharmacy Benefit
Management). *See* Pharmacy
Benefit Management
(PBM)
PeakMed Primary Care, 34–35
Peck, Ron E. *See* administrative
services
pharmaceutical industry. *See
also* Transparent Pharmacy
Benefits (TPB)
certification, 216–217
and fraud, 99–100
and physicians, 207
reporting, 213–214
sales and marketing by, 4, 12
specialty, 260
pharmacies, 228
Pharmacy Benefit Management
(PBM)
about, xx, 257

contracts, understanding,
258–259, 259f
and fraud, 99–100
incentives of, 261
and pricing, 79–80, 134, 260–261
physical therapy (PT)
and back pain, 78
insurance coverage of, 6
and overtreatment, 113–114
public sector employees, 22
in value-based primary care
(VBPC), 227
physicians. *See also* primary care
accessory, 81–82
burnout of, 30–31, 341
compensation of, 226, 343–344
and pharmaceutical industry, 207
pill mills, 8
Pittsburgh (Allegheny County)
Schools, 37–41, 170, 194, 278
Plumas County (California),
206–208
politics, and health care, 160–162.
See also nonpartisan, health
care as
polypharmacy, 214–215
portals, patient, 227
post-surgical prescribing (opioids),
213
PPOs (Preferred Provider
Organization), 50–51, 87–88,
149
premiums, insurance, 27
prenatal care, 72, 135
prescriptions. *See also*
pharmaceutical industry
certification, 216
distribution channels of, 260
volume reports (opioids),
213–214
presenteeism, 9

CPSIA information can be obtained
at www.ICGtesting.com
Printed in the USA
LVHW08s1031011018
591921LV00019B/657/P

9 780999 234334